The Language of Pain

Converging Evidence in Language and Communication Research (CELCR)

Over the past decades, linguists have taken a broader view of language and are borrowing methods and findings from other disciplines such as cognition and computer sciences, neurology, biology, sociology, psychology, and anthropology. This development has enriched our knowledge of language and communication, but at the same time it has made it difficult for researchers in a particular field of language studies to be aware of how their findings might relate to those in other (sub-)disciplines.

CELCR seeks to address this problem by taking a cross-disciplinary approach to the study of language and communication. The books in the series focus on a specific linguistic topic and offer studies pertaining to this topic from different disciplinary angles, thus taking converging evidence in language and communication research as its basic methodology.

Volume 9

The Language of Pain. Expression or description?
Chryssoula Lascaratou

The Language of Pain

Expression or description?

Chryssoula Lascaratou
University of Athens

John Benjamins Publishing Company
Amsterdam / Philadelphia

∞™ The paper used in this publication meets the minimum requirements of American National Standard for Information Sciences – Permanence of Paper for Printed Library Materials, ANSI Z39.48-1984.

Library of Congress Cataloging-in-Publication Data

Lascaratou, Chryssoula.

The Language of Pain : expression or description? / Chryssoula Lascaratou.

p. cm. -- (Converging evidence in language and communication research, ISSN 1566-7774 ; v. 9)

Includes bibliographical references and index.

1. Psycholinguistics--Data processing. 2. Pain--Data processing. 3. Lexicology--Data processing. 4. Greek language, Modern--Psychological aspects--Data processing. I. Title.

P37.5.D37L37 2007

410.1'9--dc22 2007026886

ISBN 978 90 272 3896 2 (Hb; alk. paper)

John Benjamins Publishing Co. · P.O. Box 36224 · 1020 ME Amsterdam · The Netherlands

John Benjamins North America · P.O. Box 27519 · Philadelphia PA 19118-0519 · USA *for Angelos*

Table of contents

Acknowledgements XI

CHAPTER 1
Introduction 1

CHAPTER 2
Pain and language 9
2.1 Introduction 9
2.2 The language of pain 13
2.2.1 What is pain? 14
2.2.1.1 The IASP definition and reasons for adopting it 15
2.2.1.2 Other attempts at interpreting and defining pain 16
2.2.2 What is language for pain? 19
2.2.2.1 Wittgenstein's 'private language argument' and pain 20
2.2.2.2 The function of pain language: Expressive and/or descriptive? 24
2.2.2.3 How is pain transformed into language? 27
2.2.3 What is pain for language? 28

CHAPTER 3
Corpus design and data collection 31

CHAPTER 4
Mode of analysis 37
4.1 Introduction 37
4.2 Halliday's process types in modelling experience 38

CHAPTER 5
Data analysis and general discussion 45
5.1 Introduction 45
5.2 Pain: Process, participant or quality? 45
5.3 Key lexical items and their frequencies 50

CHAPTER 6
The construal of pain as process 59
6.1 Introduction 59
6.2 Foolen's account of the communication of emotions and pain behaviour 59
6.3 General characteristics of pain as process 61
6.4 Process types and structural functions in ***ponao*** constructions 73
6.4.1 Concluding remarks 100

CHAPTER 7
The construal of pain as thing-participant 103
7.1 Introduction 103
7.2 Grammatically construed semantic properties of ***ponos*** 104
7.2.1 *Ponos* as a bounded or an unbounded thing 104
7.2.2 *Ponos* as a possession: Acquired, received, owned, and lost 106
7.2.3 The temporal location and extent of *ponos* 108
7.2.4 The accompanying conditions of *ponos*: A temporal nexus 110
7.2.5 The variable location of *ponos* within the body 111
7.2.6 The degree of intensity and the variable qualities of *ponos*: Mapping the Greek data onto the McGill Pain Questionnaire (MPQ) 113
7.2.6.1 The intensity of pain 115
7.2.6.2 The variable qualities of pain 118
7.2.7 Concluding remarks 123
7.3 Structural configurations featuring ***ponos*** as participant 124
7.3.1 Concluding remarks 132

CHAPTER 8
Pain and metaphor 133
8.1 Introduction 133
8.2 The conceptual grounding of ***ponos*** metaphors and their linguistic realisation 139
8.2.1 The grammaticalisation of *ponos* as object of the verbs *exo*, *esθanome*, and *njoθo* 140
8.2.2 The grammaticalisation of *ponos* as subject in intransitive structures 147
8.2.3 The grammaticalisation of *ponos* as subject in transitive structures 155
8.2.4 The construal of *ponos* as circumstance of cause 170
8.2.5 The grammaticalisation of *ponos* as object in transitive structures 172
8.3 Lost for words 174
8.4 Concluding remarks 178

CHAPTER 9
Conclusions 183

References 197

Appendix A: Pain as process. Mapping Greek 'pain' expressions onto Halliday's paradigm of English ones 207

Appendix B: Pain as thing. Mapping Greek 'pain' expressions onto Halliday's paradigm of English ones 215

Appendix C: Typical corpus dialogues presented in full 219
1. Private physiotherapy clinic. Dialogue No 6 219
2. Metaxa Cancer Hospital, pain management clinic. Dialogue No 17 227

Name index 233

Subject index 235

Acknowledgements

It is with great pleasure that I acknowledge my debt to the many people who offered me their help in various respects and at various stages of the preparation of this book.

I would like to express my gratitude and indebtedness to Dimitra Theophanopoulou-Kontou for her instructive comments on an earlier version of this book. I am mostly indebted and grateful to Zoltán Kövecses for carefully reading the manuscript and generously giving me so much of his time in inspiring and stimulating discussions. In particular, much of what is worthwhile in the chapter on pain and metaphor has its roots in what I learnt from him. Above all, I wish to thank Zoltán for showing interest in my work and being a constant source of encouragement, support and invaluable advice.

I would also like to express my sincere thanks to Ourania Hatzidaki not only for generously offering me her expertise in various aspects of the statistical analysis of the data and her constructive comments on related parts of the manuscript, but also for genuinely sharing my deep involvement in exploring the complexities of pain through its linguistic dimension.

Special thanks are due to many colleagues, students, and friends for their encouragement and many constructive discussions and comments. Among those, I wish to extend my thanks to Athanassios Alexandridis, Sophia Antonakaki, Bessie Dendrinos, Georgia Frangaki, Dionysis Goutsos, Elly Ifantidou, Nikos Karandreas, Sophia Marmaridou, Spiros Moschonas, Anastasia Papaconstantinou, Irene Philippaki-Warburton, Antigone Philippopoulou, Mary Sifianou, Ioannis Veloudis, and David Warburton.

I am greatly indebted to Palina Karakasidou, Georgia Petta (Department of Physiotherapy, Technological Education Institute of Athens – TEI), Stavros Stathopoulos (Physiotherapy Clinic, Evangelismos Hospital), Costas Levidiotis (Orthopedics Clinic, Evgenidio Hospital), Calliope Kastrinaki (Pain Clinic, Metaxa Cancer Hospital), Michel Amari, Katerina Harkiolaki, Yannis Paxinos (Pain Clinic, Patision General Prefectural Hospital), and Michalis Seferiadis (Physiotherapy Clinic, Patision General Prefectural Hospital) for participating in the project by supplying the recorded material. I also wish to express my sincere thanks to the students of the Faculty of English Studies (University of Athens) Panagoula Barlia, Spyridoula Dimopoulou, Dimitris Farmakis, Christina Karamouza, Maria Karteri, Constantina Kotsira, Constantina Liontou, Kyriaki Mantzarli, Eleni Mouzouraki, Efstathios Nikolopoulos, Despina Panou, Ekaterini Pappa, Paschalia Patsala, Maria Pepe, Loukia Sigala, Eleni Taratsa, Evdoksia Tsiombika and Alexandros Velaoras for transcribing the recordings. The collection and transcription of the data might not have been attained without the considerable assistance of all the above. I am also particularly indebted to Fanis Papoutsis for his valuable assistance in the preparation of Appendix C.

I would like to record my very special thanks and deepest gratitude to Michalis Georgiafentis for the patience, enthusiasm, and dedication with which he so selflessly assisted me in various aspects of this work. In particular, I am indebted to Michalis for eagerly offering his expertise and willingly devoting valuable time in sharing with me the burden of editing this work. My most whole-hearted thanks go to Dorothy Richardson for readily making the time to proof-read the whole manuscript and add an expert's final touches to the text.

On a more personal note, I would like to express my gratitude and warmest thanks to my son Angelos Aivazis for his loving support, understanding, and unique sense of humour, which made the completion of this work much more enjoyable and less painful.

This book has benefited from all those acknowledged above, but of course all inadequacies and infelicities that may remain are entirely my own. Finally, I wish to apologise to anyone I have inadvertently omitted.

CHAPTER 1

Introduction

This book is the outcome of a long-term, large-scale, data-based investigation of the linguistic manifestation of physical pain in Modern Greek. The linguistic patterning (lexico-phraseological choices, grammatical structures, and linguistic metaphors) of pain is investigated by observing how pain is talked about in a specialised, coherent and intensively studied electronic corpus of 131 spontaneous dialogues (69,996 words) between pain-suffering patients and health care professionals, recorded over a period of 22 months. Drawing on tools widely used for corpus analysis, a combined qualitative and quantitative methodology is applied.

My interest in studying the linguistic dimension of pain, as a domain of human experience lying at the intersection of the physical and psychological aspects of our selves, emerged quite naturally from my intense preoccupation with the relation between body, soul, and language over the past decade. Pain language as a research area became even more challenging to me when my bibliographical exploration revealed that it had not as yet been systematically investigated from a purely linguistic perspective either within or across languages, with the exception of Halliday's (1998) functional account of English pain expressions. Hence, I was confronted with the challenge of launching the linguistic study of the construal of pain in Greek and, thus, significantly contributing to the development of this research domain with data from a language other than English.

The crucial questions addressed by Halliday concerning the nature of the lexicogrammatical construal of pain (i.e. as process, participant, quality or circumstance) played a central part in conceiving the present study. One of my basic hypotheses is that the degree of involvement of the sufferer's self in the painful experience is a fundamental factor determining the character of its linguistic framing.

Halliday's proposed paradigm provided me with the necessary theoretical ground, within the broader framework of Functional Grammar. Moreover, in the analysis of the role of metaphor in conceptualising and representing pain, a cognitive semantics perspective was adopted (Kövecses 1990, 1995, 2000, 2005, forth.; Lakoff and Johnson, 1999; and Talmy, 1988, among others), which complements the functional account, the two approaches essentially converging in some basic aspects of their interpretation of this experiential domain, as will be shown in the relevant parts of this study. The points of contact between the two models, as was initially claimed in Lascaratou and Marmaridou (2005: 235), may be related to their methodological compatibility, i.e. that in both models language is viewed as *construing* human experience rather than *objectively reflecting* reality, the former prioritising "the role of lexico-grammar in construing reality, whereas the latter typically emphasises the conceptual mechanisms that motivate such construals." Hence, as will be argued in various parts of the data analysis, there are cases where these two different usage-based approaches seem to converge, to complement each other, in an interesting manner, the insights expressed through the functional paradigm being conceptually grounded in the cognitive semantic approach. In other words, on various occasions a cognitive semantic interpretation of the data will provide a justification for their functional account.

In the light of Wittgenstein's (1953/1989) understanding of the role of ordinary language in publicly communicating pain (i.e. his 'private language' concept) and on the basis of my authentic doctor-patient Greek data and my native speaker's intuitions, I shall engage in the investigation of the framing of pain in Greek, by analysing its lexico-grammatical characteristics. The 'cartography' of pain that I shall attempt will reveal the variety of roles played by pain configurations in transforming pain into meaning in our everyday lives. My analysis will revolve around the sufferer – as the centre of the experience – and his multiple construals as Actor, Carrier, Experiencer, Goal, Senser, etc. vis-à-vis the painful experience itself with its multiple construals as Goal, Attribute, Phenomenon, Medium, Existent, etc.

The analysis proposed is motivated by Halliday's (1998) claim about the fundamental role of lexico-grammar in construing our everyday experience semantically, i.e. in conceptualising our world in general. Thus, from his functional perspective, Halliday sees lexico-grammar as the energetic core of language and argues that its power stems from the fact that grammar is the source of energy for our everyday experience. More specifically, Halliday (*ibid.*: 30) accounts for the power that we proclaim language to have in social and political life in terms of its ability to systematise our everyday encounters with the world:

> enabling us to talk about them to each other, giving them value, and so helping us to 'make sense' of things that we still, for all our cleverness, cannot control.

In my mode of analysis, I am essentially adopting Gustafson's (1979: 151–152) suggestion about how researchers typically proceed with the investigation of an object of inquiry: they first carry out a grammatical analysis so as to gain some insights into its nature and provide an initial answer to the question "*what* kind of thing it is." On the basis of their preliminary findings, they then proceed to the next step, which is to further elaborate and refine their research on a level of increased specificity so as to reveal the various aspects of their object of investigation, i.e. provide a detailed answer to the question "*which* kind this kind is."

Thus, by identifying the predominant character of pain as process, participant or quality in the first place, and then thoroughly studying the various structural configurations whereby pain is construed linguistically, I aim at providing an understanding of how the Greek language profiles pain in everyday encounters. This inquiry will allow me to achieve the ultimate goal of the present study, which is to answer in an empirically verifiable way the question concerning the function of language in the experience of pain (see Gustafson, 1979; Kenny, 1973; Kripke, 1982; Wittgenstein, 1953/1989): is its function that of expression or description, or both, and which one is primary? Moreover, is it the case that under certain circumstances language does not prove to be rich enough to encode the sufferer's subjective, private, unpleasant condition?

Ultimately, by making pain our *object* of research, we are unconsciously (or subconsciously) engaging ourselves in a process of *objectifying* it, thus, coming face to face with it so as to accept its universality and perhaps tame "this arbitrary and ruthless enemy" that "lurks and strikes apparently at random" (Halliday, 1998: 29).

Before moving on to a presentation of the structure of the book, it is worth noting here that as part of my long-term, large-scale, corpus-based investigation, two articles comprising preliminary surveys have already emerged. Both articles, namely, Lascaratou and Hatzidaki (2002) – a first taxonomy of pain-related lexico-phraseological forms and syntactic structures – and Lascaratou and Marmaridou (2005) – an initial account of the conceptual basis of metaphorical pain language – are based on the analysis of a subcorpus of my material, i.e. 85 authentic doctor-patient dialogues (47,464 words) that I collected at an early stage of the research project. In addition to this subcorpus-corpus relation between the data of the two articles and those of the present study, the preliminary surveys have served the purpose of providing the necessary testing ground for the analysis and interpretation of the data observed in the extensive corpus of my research project. The early brief analyses are followed up in this book in terms of more comprehensive and elaborate accounts, where both a wider range of linguistic patterns is thoroughly examined and the analytical tools are considerably refined. Hence, the original insights are more firmly grounded, while new claims are more confidently voiced.

Thus, in Lascaratou and Hatzidaki (2002), Halliday's (1998) functional account of English pain expressions is first employed as the theoretical framework for a preliminary analysis of only the four most frequently occurring Greek *ponao*

'I hurt' verb patterns.[1] From that early analysis, one of the central claims of the research project – further reinforced in this book against additional data – clearly emerges: it is suggested that, in everyday encounters, Greek construes pain primarily as an intransitive personal 'process' and secondarily as 'participant', with the body part only rarely being construed as the locus of pain. A subsequent elaborate account of this initially observed intransitive character of pain configurations and of the holistic understanding of pain is to be found in Chapter 6.

As for the second article, it was originally motivated by my observation that, quite often, the patients in the dialogues collected actually use metaphorical language to talk about their pain, an observation already put forward in the social sciences and psychology literature (e.g. Aldrich and Eccleston, 2000; Kugelmann, 1999; Söderberg and Norberg, 1995). Hence, in Lascaratou and Marmaridou (2005) the focus is on *ponos* 'pain' nominal constructions and their metaphorical motivation, the original functional framework being complemented by a cognitive perspective (Lakoff and Johnson, 1999 and Talmy, 1988, among others) for an initial exploration of the conceptual structure of pain. This theoretical 'toolbox', where two different – yet converging – usage-based approaches are combined, has been extensively used in the data analysis of the present study, with interesting overlaps between the Hallidayan and cognitive semantic treatments being traced. Moreover, the early account of the conceptual basis of pain language is followed up in Chapter 8: on the grounds of a modified application of Talmy's (1988) force dynamic schema, and drawing on Kövecses's (2000 and forth.) analysis of metaphor and emotion (and its application to the conceptual structure of pain), a revised analysis is proposed in terms of the master metaphor PAIN IS A FORCE.

In addition to this introduction, the book comprises eight chapters and three appendices.

In Chapter 2 the linguistic dimension of pain is introduced. It is pointed out that, despite the rising interest in the study of the language of emotions over the past twenty years, there has not been any systematic analysis of the language of pain so far, although pain is undoubtedly related to emotions through its widely acknowledged emotional aspect. The currently accepted definition of pain, as recommended by the International Association for the Study of Pain (IASP), is presented and reasons are provided for adopting it as a working definition. The complexity of this experiential domain is brought out by reference to some of its

1. All Greek data are presented in broad phonemic transcription, with the use of the characters of the Latin alphabet. In addition, the Greek characters γ, δ, θ are used to represent the phonemes /ɣ/ (voiced velar fricative), /ð/ (voiced dental fricative), and /θ/ (voiceless dental fricative), respectively. A word-by-word (or morpheme-by-morpheme, where necessary) gloss is provided, followed by a free translation into English.

fundamental attributes, as these are treated in various approaches, e.g. medical, neuroscience, psychoanalytic. The relation of language to pain is then brought in and its subtleties are discussed in the light of Wittgenstein's philosophical 'private language' argument. The question as to whether pain utterances are primarily expressions or descriptions of the sensation is crucially posed, and it is suggested that, in attempting to provide an answer, its grammatical representation should be thoroughly considered. Hence, the significance attributed to lexico-grammar by Halliday in conceptualising our world is endorsed and the need to investigate the grammatical construal of pain in an attempt to gain a better understanding of this inevitable human experience is put forward.

In Chapter 3 the reasons underlying my decision to collect a corpus of authentic dialogues between pain-suffering patients and medical experts are exposed. Thus, it is argued that the subjectivity, complexity and diversity of physical pain make it imperative to look into utterances spontaneously produced by a considerable number of sufferers, rather than rely on personal intuitions and observations alone. Details of the corpus design and the data collection are presented as well as the material and its sources.

Chapter 4 initiates the reader into Halliday's understanding of the 'experiential' function of the clause in terms of processes (e.g. 'happening', 'doing', 'sensing', 'meaning', and 'being and becoming') within Functional Grammar. This brief account of the theoretical model adopted in this study is necessary for the presentation and functional interpretation of the observed Greek data and their juxtaposition with Halliday's paradigm of English pain expressions in the subsequent chapters.

Chapter 5 presents a characterisation of the lexico-grammatical construal of pain in Greek, on the basis of frequency counts applied on the findings. Thus, on the grounds of empirical evidence emerging from the doctor-patient dialogues, it is claimed that in Greek the framing of pain is primarily verbal (denoting a process), secondarily nominal (denoting a participant), and only marginally adjectival (denoting a quality). Assuming that the lexico-grammatical construal of pain is related to the degree of involvement of the sufferer's self in the painful experience, an initial interpretation of the observed predominantly verbal framing of pain along the lines of Wierzbicka's (1992) account of the construction of emotions is put forward, to be taken up in a more thorough discussion in Chapter 6. This first picture of the linguistic representation of pain is complemented by the identification of some of the recurrent key lexical items observed in the doctor-patient discourse of pain.

The processual construal of pain in terms of the various patterns of the *ponao* 'I hurt' verb paradigm observed in the naturally-occurring data is examined in Chapter 6. All eight structures collected in the corpus are discussed in detail and interpreted in terms of the different types of figure (i.e. 'doing and happening', 'sensing' and 'being') into which pain as process enters, as well as in terms of the functions assigned to the participants and to the sufferer, in particular (e.g. Carrier, Actor, Senser, Goal, etc.). The analysis focuses mainly on the two most frequent of the eight collected structures, namely, the intransitive-personal *ponao* 'I hurt' / 'I'm hurting' (46.82%) and the intransitive-impersonal *ponai* 'it hurts' / 'it's hurting' (19.66%), their interpretation requiring reference to both their experiential grammar and the textual component of grammar. Thus, it is suggested that the chiefly intransitive quality of the verbal framing of pain can be interpreted as a special grammatical property whereby the understanding of pain as an inner activity or a self-induced processual event is more vividly brought out. In addition, it is proposed that the statistical dominance of intransitive *ponao* avowals and *ponai* utterances can also be accounted for in terms of the superiority of intransitive verbs over multi-argument structures with respect to their ability to represent a more 'primitive' form of voicing automatic reactions. As for the locus of pain, it is observed that in the great majority (56.66%) of its processual construals pain is configured holistically, i.e. as dwelling in the sufferer's self as a whole rather than in a body part. This holistic thematic perspective from which the painful sensation is presented is mainly created through *ponao* 'I hurt' / 'I'm hurting' avowals. Finally, the analysis of the diverse processual configurations of pain in Greek reveals that, on the whole, these have a stronger expressive rather than descriptive function. In particular, it is suggested that certain instances of intransitive first-person *ponao* 'I hurt' / 'I'm hurting' or impersonal third-person *ponai* 'it hurts' / 'it's hurting' pain utterances can be identified with a potential direct linguistic expression of pain and, hence, they should be placed in positions adjacent to those of interjections and automatic non-linguistic pain reactions (e.g. cries / groans / screams) along the expressive-descriptive axis of the proposed continuum. The assumed gradience of the expressive function is schematically represented by symbolically arranging the remaining patterns in intermediate positions.

Chapter 7 comprises a thorough lexico-grammatical analysis of pain as thing, linguistically realised in Greek by *ponos* nominal expressions, in terms of the seven grammatically construed semantic features of pain proposed by Halliday (1998), e.g. its construal as a possession, its variable intensity, qualities and location within the body. On the basis of the analysis of the doctor-patient data, it is claimed that the validity of these features, as dimensions along which the painful experience can be made an 'object' of description, measurement and assessment, may confidently be extended to Greek. Along the lines of Halliday's paradigm of 'pain as thing', the observed structural configurations are then analysed in terms of the process types into which *ponos* enters as a participant (i.e. 'doing', 'sensing', and 'being and having') and the structural functions assigned to pain (e.g. Goal, Phenomenon, Carrier, Attribute, Existent, etc.). The observation that nowhere in this paradigm does pain bear the transitive function of Actor or the ergative function of (external) Agent, even though it may appear grammaticalised as the subject in a structure, is of vital importance for the analysis. The descriptive character of *ponos* nominal constructions, emerging from the functional analysis of their lexico-grammatical properties, is even more vividly brought to light when we move to metaphorically structured expressions and approach them from a cognitive semantics perspective (e.g. Kövecses 1990, 1995, 2000, 2005, forth.; Lakoff and Johnson, 1999; and Talmy, 1988) in the next chapter.

Chapter 8 deals with the role of metaphor in conceptualising pain in everyday encounters. The Greek doctor-patient data lend support to the view often expressed that metaphorical pain language is typically associated with the inherent difficulty of describing, i.e. communicating, this complex, invisible, private sensation. With *ponos* nominal constructions in focus and from a cognitive semantics perspective, it is argued that the pain-related data provide empirical evidence in support of the view that the linguistic realisation of metaphors and the selection of particular lexical frames are motivated by image schematic conceptual structure, while conceptualisations of everyday experience are shaped by linguistic structure, i.e. by language-specific syntactico-semantic constraints. In particular, the data analysis consistently highlights the close relation between the metaphorical representation of pain and the constraints imposed by the grammaticalisation of *ponos* as syntactic object (e.g. of the possessive verb *exo* 'have') – whereby it gains distance and independence from the sufferer – or as subject of intransitive verbs (e.g. of motion) and, above all, of transitive ones. The exploitation of the animacy feature of certain configurations leads to a number of very closely related conceptualisations in which *ponos* appears, *inter alia*, as A SELF-WILLED INTRUSIVE and MALEVOLENT AGGRESSOR, A RUTHLESS TORTURER, AN IMPRISONING ENEMY. On the basis of Talmy's (1988) force dynamic schema and in the light of Kövecses (2000 and forth.), it is argued that the specific-level pain metaphors observed in the Greek data are instantiations of such a general metaphor as PAIN IS A FORCE. Such metaphorical construals of pain, which appear to be chiefly focusing on the cause of the sensation, are shown to be also motivated and maintained by doctor-patient discourse practices. Crucially, the concept of 'embodiment' is invoked to account for the constraints imposed on the cognitive mechanisms (conceptual metonymies and metaphors) underlying Greek pain metaphors by the universal aspects of the human body's physiology in pain (various types of tissue damage with their accompanying sensory effects). To conclude, it is argued that when pain is communicated by means of *ponos* objectifying constructions, in particular metaphorically motivated descriptions, the role of pain utterances is undoubtedly descriptive. Such metaphorical structures, therefore, should feature on the extreme pole representing the descriptive function in the suggested schematic continuum of pain manifestations.

In Chapter 9 the most important conclusions of this long-term study are put forward.

Appendices A (pain as process) and B (pain as thing) schematically present Greek pain expressions as analysed in this study along the lines of Halliday's paradigm. Finally, in Appendix C two typical corpus dialogues are presented in full.

CHAPTER 2

Pain and language

2.1 Introduction

The complex, private, central and ubiquitous experience of pain, an essential and inevitable part of the human condition, is characterised by different physical, psychological and socio-cultural aspects. In Kugelmann's words (1999: 1663), "Pain in its expression, alleviation and suffering, is a performance that is as personal as cultural, as mental as bodily: Just as the making of love."

Due precisely to its multi-dimensional character, pain has been investigated from various perspectives: it has primarily been the object of scrutiny from a medical perspective (e.g. Ashburn and Rice, 1998; Borsook, LeBel and McPeek, 1998; Melzack, 1975; Melzack and Torgerson, 1971; Melzack and Wall, 1988; Wall and Melzack (eds), 1989), but also from a psychological, anthropological, philosophical and historical perspective (e.g. Aldrich and Eccleston, 2000; Baszanger, 1992; Del Vecchio Good et al., 1992; Foucault, 1991; Jackson, 1992, 1994; Kleinman, 1988, 1996; Kugelmann, 1999; Levinas, 1988, 1991; Morris, 1991; Rey, 1993/1998; Scarry, 1985; Schweizer, 1995; Toombs, 1993; Waddie, 1996; Wittgenstein, 1953/1989).

Pain also presents a linguistic dimension. However, despite the central role of language in human pain behaviour, for linguists, pain has not as yet been the object of comprehensive study within and across languages. Thus, though there are some very insightful accounts of pain language, these are mainly based on experiments on pain expressions and terms used by patients and medical / nursing staff with a view to measuring and assessing pain (e.g. Edwards and Pearce, 1994; Fabrega and Tyma, 1976a, 1976b; Gaston-Johansson, 1984; Georgoudis, Watson and Oldham, 2000; Georgoudis, Oldham and Watson, 2001; Janal, 1995; Norvell, Gaston-Johansson and Zimmerman, 1990; Papageorgiou and Badley, 1989; Pincus, Pearce and Perrott, 1996; Söderberg and Norberg, 1995). That is, they are not purely linguistic studies but rather they have either a medical, psychological or a social science orientation, their primary aim being to provide medical and social science experts with useful insights into the experience of pain mainly for the elaboration of medical or psychological treatments and social policies.

The absence of linguistic studies on the verbal dimension of pain is striking, given that over the last two decades there has been an increasing interest in the study of a closely related domain, namely, the language of emotions. The relation between language and emotion has been the object of linguistic analysis from a rather wide range of perspectives.[1] The way language is linked to emotion in a particular approach is determined by how emotion is viewed within it (Pavlenko, 2002: 208–211).

The widely accepted Darwinian view that there exists a basic set of biologically predetermined universal human emotions underlies the neuroscience approach of LeDoux (1998) and Damasio (1999) who propose that emotions evolved as brain states and bodily responses which belong to our bio-regulatory equipment by means of which we survive. This universalist approach to emotion also essentially underlies the psychological work of Izard (1977, 1992) and Ekman (1980, 1992, 1993) who argue for a finite set of basic universal human emotions such as anger, disgust, enjoyment, fear, sadness, and shame which correspond to these particular English words and are claimed to be uniformly mirrored in all languages and unvaryingly identifiable cross-culturally. It follows that the universalist perspective entails a separatist view of language and emotion: language (understood in the broadest sense) and (the expression of) emotions are viewed as "two concurrent, parallel systems, in use" (Bamberg, 1997: 209), "whereby one system (emotions) may impact the performance of another (language)" (Pavlenko, 2002: 208). Within this perspective, in order to gain insights into the mechanisms of the emotional mind, researchers conduct studies using "verbal stimuli as the gateway to emotions or verbal reports to measure emotions" (LeDoux, 1998: 71).

However, in the last two decades, the domain of emotions has become the object of research not only in separate studies in psychology, philosophy, sociology, ethnology, and linguistics, but mainly in studies conducted by researchers following an interdisciplinary approach, such as cultural psychologists, social constructionists, linguistic anthropologists, and cognitive linguists (e.g. Athanasiadou and Tabakowska (eds), 1998; Kövecses 1990, 1995, 2000, 2005, forth.; Niemeier and Dirven (eds), 1997; Enfield and Wierzbicka (eds), 2002 (*Pragmatics and Cognition* 10 (1–2), special issue on *The Body in Description of Emotion: Cross-Linguistic Studies*); Wierzbicka, 1980, 1988, 1992, 1995a, 1996, 1997, 1999). In these endeavours the separatist view of language and emotion entailed in the universalist approach is criticised and language is understood as being closely and dynamically linked to

1. To mention but a few, lexicographic research on emotion words is to be found in such works as Solomon (1995), Wierzbicka (1995b), and Omondi (1997), emotion verbs are analysed syntactically in Nissenbaum (1985), the 'pragmatics of affect' are dealt with in a special issue of the *Journal of Pragmatics* (1994), vol. 22 (3/4) and, most importantly, the way languages conceptualise emotions is studied within the framework of cognitive semantics (see below).

emotion and cognition, so that it "no longer 'mirrors' the world of emotions but instead actively constructs and reconstructs it" (Pavlenko, 2002: 209). Hence, great significance is attributed to language "in the quest to understand cognitive aspects of emotion and other social phenomena" (Enfield and Wierzbicka, 2002: 7). Research chiefly focuses on the aspect of cognition involved in conceptualising emotion experience through linguistic categories (words, constructions). (For a psychoanalytically oriented semantic treatment of emotions, where some of the basic assumptions of cognitive linguistics are challenged, see Theodoropoulou, 1999, 2004, forth.) Consequently, the study of the language of emotions is becoming increasingly central in the research domain of emotions, with the issue of what constitutes emotional meaning, i.e. what the meaning of emotion words and terms is composed of, being "a hotly debated topic in several disciplines – from psychology through anthropology to philosophy" (Kövecses 2000: 6).

Thus, for example, from a cognitive semantics perspective, Wierzbicka (1992, 1997) assumes that emotional meaning consists of universal semantic primitives: conceptual primitives, combined in certain ways, make up the conceptual content of particular emotion words in particular languages.[2] She suggests that emotions are differently conceptualised across different languages and cultures. Every language is assumed to impose its own classification upon human emotional experiences, in terms of its own set of ready-made emotion words designating those emotions that are recognised as particularly salient in a given culture. On the other hand, she convincingly argues (1992: 124), though the evidence available suggests that there are no emotion concepts which have been *lexically* recognised as distinct and identifiable in all languages of the world, she does not wish to rule out the possibility that there are some *psychologically* distinct and clearly identifiable universal human emotions, or at least pan-human emotional prototypes. Such

2. For Wierzbicka (1992: 178), the concept of 'emotion' involves "a combination of 'feeling', 'thinking', and an unspecified internal process" which, in the language of universal semantic primitives, could be represented as follows:

> *emotion*
> person X thought something
> because of this, X felt something
> because of this, something happened to X

Thus, Wierzbicka's research is based on her assumption that emotions are both cognitive and physiological, rather than purely 'biological events', and involve "someone *feeling* something in the context of their *thinking* something" (see Enfield and Wierzbicka, 2002: 4). On the other hand, in her anthropological account, Rosaldo (1984: 143), as reported in Enfield and Wierzbicka (2002: 6), identifies emotions as "thoughts somehow 'felt' in flushes, pulses, 'movements' of our livers, minds, hearts, stomachs, skin." Notably, Wierzbicka deals with the conceptualising function of language, not its expressive function, the study of the latter within the framework of cognitive semantics having been first explored by Foolen (1997) as 'expressive semantics'.

universal emotions, she maintains (correctly, I think), "cannot be identified by means of English folk categories such as *anger*, *shame*, or *disgust*; they can only be identified in a culture-independent semantic metalanguage" (*ibid.*: 176).[3] Hence, within the so-called Natural Semantic Metalanguage (NSM) framework, Wierzbicka calls for a maximally culture-free, language-independent, cross-linguistic perspective in identifying and mapping universal human emotions that have not been widely lexicalised in different languages.[4]

The essence of Wierzbicka's cognitive semantic approach to emotions and their relation to language and culture is reflected in the following lines which reveal her understanding of (conceptual and linguistic) universals and the importance she attributes to empirical data:

> Crucially, from our point of view, sound semantic analysis must be anchored in empirically attested conceptual and linguistic universals. [...] Without some such universals – that is without a set of shared concepts which can be used as maximally culture independent analytical tools – the conceptualisation of emotions across languages and cultures could never be precisely and effectively compared: there can be no effective comparison without a *tertium comparationis* (Enfield and Wierzbicka, 2002: 7).

Wierzbicka's proposed NSM, or 'universal language of thought', consisting of universal primitive concepts to be applied for the description and comparison of meanings – including emotional meaning – across languages, is very insightful

3. Wierzbicka considers such emotion words to be mere labels, i.e. cultural artefacts, of the English language, not necessarily corresponding to feelings expressed by similar labels in other languages. She, therefore, essentially argues against the ethnocentricity underlying Ekman's view that universal emotions are identifiable on the basis of such English terms.

4. The fundamental assumption (or working hypothesis) on which Wierzbicka's work is based is that all languages have an innate common core (both in their lexicons and in their grammar) which is being "shaped by a prelinguistic 'readiness for meaning'" (Wierzbicka, 1997: 24). Most importantly, this presumed common core "is determined by an innate conceptual system, and it is independent of everything idiosyncratic in the structure of all individual languages" (*ibid.* 1997: 24). The assumed conceptual primitives, together with certain innate and universal rules of syntax, which are hypothesised to determine possible combinations of primitive concepts, make up 'a language of thought', or *Lingua Mentalis* (Wierzbicka, 1980), which is proposed as a practical, culture-free, natural semantic metalanguage (NSM) to be employed for the description and comparison of meanings across languages.

and attractive as an abstract theoretical system.[5] However, though its application in the domain of emotions may yield adequate accounts of many aspects of emotional meaning, it seems that the contribution of such conceptual mechanisms as metaphor and metonymy in the understanding of emotion concepts is not considered. In my analysis of the metaphorical representation of pain (see Chapter 8), therefore, I will adopt a cognitive semantics perspective (e.g. Kövecses 1990, 1995, 2000, 2005, forth.; Lakoff and Johnson, 1999; and Talmy, 1988) in which it is claimed that metaphor plays a central role in the conceptualisation of human experience in general and of emotions, in particular. Moreover, in the approach I will follow, certain aspects of the human body are assumed to play an important role in the conceptualisation of emotions: fundamental bodily experiences motivate certain basic image schemas which are claimed to be universal, while universal human physiology largely constrains the metaphorical representation of emotions.

2.2 The language of pain

Though, as it will be shown later on in our discussion of the definition of pain, this private sensation is not identified as an emotion in the strict sense in which such psychological experiences as fear, anger, shame, sadness, disgust and enjoyment are, yet the emotional aspect of the experience of pain is widely accepted as one of its fundamental dimensions. (See section 2.2.1.1 below for a presentation and analysis of the definition provided by the International Association for the Study of Pain (IASP) where pain is explicitly identified as also being an emotional experience, by virtue of being unpleasant.) It is surprising, therefore, that alongside the study of 'the language of emotions', there has not been any systematic analysis of 'the language of pain' so far. It is noteworthy, however, that even with respect to the language of emotions the need for more systematic linguistic investigation has been voiced: "the desideratum of theoretically sound research of both the lexicon and the grammar of emotions from a single-language or a cross-linguistic perspective remains" (Niemeier, 1997: ix). The motivation underlying research on the language of emotions as expressed in Enfield and Wierzbicka's claim (2002: 2), namely, that it is impossible to explore "other people's emotions without keeping

5. Devising a workable and effective NSM to be used as a descriptive tool in wide-ranging cross-cultural semantic analysis has been a long-term, gradual process, involving successive versions based on revisions and expansions of the originally postulated (short) list of primitives, in response to empirical evidence from diverse natural languages. Hence, although a theoretically appealing and challenging hypothesis, in practice Wierzbicka's proposed NSM appears to be far from straightforward and simple to construct, if one judges from the inadequacies of its successive versions.

language in focus: both as an object and as a tool of study", equally applies to the study of the language of such an essentially private experience as pain.

To my knowledge, until recently, the only systematic linguistic account of the construal of pain by language was to be found in Halliday (1998), where a paradigm of English pain expressions is proposed from the standpoint of transitivity.[6] This functional account has served as the initial theoretical framework (later complemented by a cognitive semantic component) of my large-scale, corpus-based investigation. As was noted earlier in the introductory chapter, on the basis of the analysis of a subset of my corpus data, two preliminary surveys have already appeared, i.e. Lascaratou and Hatzidaki (2002) and Lascaratou and Marmaridou (2005), each one exploring a different aspect of the linguistic patterns of pain. (For a brief presentation of these accounts, see Chapter 1 Introduction.)

The questions that naturally arise in a study which proposes to shed light on the verbal expression of pain are:

a. What is pain?
b. What is language for pain?
c. What is pain for language?

To attempt an answer to the question *What is language for pain?* my long-term investigation presented in this study has primarily revolved around the question *What is pain for language?* To gain a better understanding of how the three questions posed above are interrelated, it seems necessary at this point to start by briefly considering how the first two have been treated.

2.2.1 What is pain?

How is pain defined? What is its nature? Is it a physical, i.e. sensory, or a psychological, i.e. emotional, event? Is it a private or a public experience?

6. In a quite recent study in the field of English historical semantics, Hans Peters (2004) attempts a preliminary analysis of the vocabulary used to talk about the concept of (physical and mental) PAIN in the history of English and of the cognitive categories and processes intrinsically linked with the semantic changes in this lexical field. As we will see in our analysis of the metaphorical representation of pain in Greek *ponos* nominal constructions (Chapter 8), there are some interesting parallels with Peters's proposed types of conceptualisation determining the way pain is talked about in English, namely, (a) PAIN IS A HOSTILE AGENT / AN ENEMY OR TORTURER causing the sensation and (b) the experience of pain is related to the CONTAINER metaphor. In a more recent study drawing on the insights of Systemic Functional Grammar, Bacchini (forth.) examines how an Italian female chronic pain sufferer makes specific lexico-grammatical choices to construct a preferred image of self. In particular, the notion of *agency* is invoked to consider how the Italian speaker positions herself vis-à-vis her illness.

According to Melzack and Torgerson (1971: 58), "the word 'pain' represents a category of experiences, signifying a multitude of different, unique events having different causes and characterized by different qualities varying along a number of sensory and affective dimensions." Thus, they define pain in terms of a multidimensional space comprising those subjective experiences which have a bodily component and produce behaviour aimed at making the conditions that produce them inoperative.

2.2.1.1 *The IASP definition and reasons for adopting it*

The currently accepted definition of pain, recommended in 1979 by the International Association for the Study of Pain (IASP), has provided researchers with a brief, yet rigorously phrased, and comprehensive answer concerning the complex nature of pain: "An unpleasant sensory and emotional experience associated with actual or potential tissue damage, or described in terms of such damage."[7]

Back in 1963 Walters, as reported in Merskey (1994: S74), had claimed that bodily pain should not be identified with its physical side – the sense data – but rather with the perceptual experience of discomfort in a spot in the body, which is a private subjective experience. Along the same lines, the IASP definition, which is based on an earlier definition originally devised by Merskey in 1964, essentially specifies that "pain [...] is always a psychological state, even though we may well appreciate that pain most often has an approximate physical cause" (Merskey, 1994: S74). Hence, according to the IASP, pain, which is always subjective, is unquestionably defined as a bodily sensation which is also always unpleasant and therefore it is also an emotional experience.

Assuming the subjective nature of pain, the IASP proposes that any experience reported in the same way as pain caused by actual tissue damage should also be accepted as pain. It therefore avoids tying pain to the stimulus and suggests that pain may be induced by any cause, including psychological ones, and that the latter will resemble the pain we first experience from physical causes "*but that it need not depend upon them*" (Merskey, 1994: S75). In essence, the IASP definition suggests that the experience of pain is largely indistinguishable by cause.

Thus, it seems that, despite its rigour, this definition allows for different interpretations, by virtue of the duality of pain involved in it, namely, its sensory-emotional aspect. It is precisely because of both its rigour and the allowances it makes that the IASP definition lends itself as a primitive in the present linguistic analysis.

7. It could be argued that the concept defined here is treated as being universal on the basis of the English word 'pain'. Yet, as in the case of other assumed universal concepts (e.g. emotion and colour), the question remains as to whether there exists a word for 'pain' as defined by the IASP in every language and culture.

In this study, which centres upon the sufferer and the diverse linguistic patterns whereby he communicates his private experience, it seemed necessary to adopt as our working definition of pain one that would not only describe it in scientific terms but also expressly bring out its subjective nature. The IASP definition, by means of the key words 'unpleasant', 'emotional', and 'potential', clearly satisfies this requirement. What is more, the subjective representation of pain is further emphasised by means of the assumption that it is essentially the sufferer who decides what pain is, since any sensation he simply 'describes' in terms of actual or potential tissue damage should be accepted as pain. In addition, this definition captures the complexity involved in the experience of pain, by assuming that it is unquestionably both a sensation and an emotional experience by virtue of being unpleasant.

On the other hand, I wish to point out that alongside the IASP *scientific definition* of pain adopted in this study, my *personal attitude* toward this subjective, private, inner sensation is best expressed in McCaffery's (1972) much quoted insightful statement, that "pain is whatever the experiencing person says it is, existing whenever he says it does."

It is worth noting here that I do not share Fabrega and Tyma's view that pain should not be defined too rigorously in a linguistic or cultural approach to pain. To be more specific, before the IASP definition was recommended, Fabrega and Tyma (1976b) decided to adopt a much broader one in their very influential study on cultural and linguistic aspects of pain, namely, that "pain is an unpleasant perception which the individual explicitly refers to his body and which can represent a form of suffering" (*ibid.*: 349). In their definition, emphasis is given to affective-motivational properties, i.e. "the perception, unpleasantness and the individual's judgment that his body or physical apparatus is the site and proximal source of the 'pain.'" Hence, the purely physiological or neurological factors are minimised, which Fabrega and Tyma, interestingly, justify by suggesting that such factors would have a negative restrictive effect on their basic aim, which is to shed light on the cultural and linguistic dimension of pain. Given that the IASP definition will not actually be applied to the data in any strict, evaluative sense but, rather, it will be assumed as a theoretical tool in our analysis, I believe that the concerns voiced by Fabrega and Tyma should not preoccupy us.

2.2.1.2 *Other attempts at interpreting and defining pain*

From a neuroscience perspective, Damasio (1999: 71) argues that pain does not qualify for emotion. That is, he does not identify the pain sensation with accompanying emotions, but suggests that both the sensation and the emotions can be caused by the same stimulus. In his own words, pain is "the consequence of a stimulus – impending or actual tissue damage – which causes the sensation of pain but also causes regulatory responses such as reflexes and may also induce emotions on its own." He also notes that pain and associated emotions are related in terms of bi-directional causation, namely, "pain can induce emotions, and some emotions can induce a state of pain" (*ibid.*: 55).

The fact that, despite its inherently internal and invisible nature, pain is also characterised by external, visible manifestations is captured in Damasio's neuroscience approach in terms of the distinction between the inward direction of the pain sensation and the outward direction of potentially accompanying regulatory reactions inducing emotions. More specifically, extending Damasio's account of emotions to pain-induced emotional responses, one can argue for the relative publicness of reactions such as changes in facial expression and posture, on the one hand, and the complete privacy of the engendered feelings, on the other. Thus, according to Damasio (*ibid.*: 36–37), emotions are outwardly directed and designate the collection of responses, many of which are publicly observable, whereas feelings (of emotions) are inwardly directed and represent the private, mental experience of an emotion. He argues that "you cannot observe a feeling in someone else although you can observe a feeling in yourself when, as a conscious being, you perceive your own emotional states. Likewise no one can observe your own feelings, but some aspects of the emotions that give rise to your feelings will be patently observable to others" (*ibid.*: 42).

Though of a different nature, a distinction between internal and external aspects of pain is also to be found in Freud's psychoanalytic treatment of pain, in terms of the internalisation of external stimuli. Thus, (physical) pain is understood as resulting in those cases where "an external stimulus becomes internal, for example by eating into and destroying a bodily organ, so that a new source of constant excitation and increase of tension is formed." The stimulus thereby functions as a pseudo-instinct, whose aim is simply "the cessation of the change in the organ and of the pain accompanying it" (Freud, 1915a/1956: 84–85). The more general perspective from which pain is viewed in this approach is that it is a regular reaction occurring "whenever a stimulus which impinges on the periphery breaks through the devices of the protective shield against stimuli and proceeds to act like a continuous instinctual stimulus, against which muscular action, which is as a rule effective because it withdraws the place that is being stimulated from the stimulus, is powerless" (Freud, 1926: 331).

The concept of *repression* also becomes central in the psychoanalytic understanding of the operation of pain: it is the state that an impulse may pass into so as to become inoperative in order for pain to be avoided. This concept allows Freud to draw a significant distinction between the idea pertaining to the repressed instinct and another element representing the instinct, which also undergoes repression but of quite a different sort from that of the idea. This leads us to that aspect of Freud's account that mainly interests our discussion of the observable dimension of pain. Namely, by means of the term *charge* (or *quota*) *of affect*, Freud expressly distinguishes that part of the instinct which has become observable to perception as *affects*, i.e. it has become detached from the idea and finds expression in processes which are sensed as affects (see Freud, 1915a/1956: 91 and 1915b/1984: 152). Thus, affects or emotions correspond "to processes of discharge, the final manifestations of which are perceived as feelings" (Freud, 1915c/1984: 181).

Within the psychoanalytic perspective, it is the relation of affects or emotions, on the one hand, and the unconscious on the other, that highlights the relation between pain and the unconscious. For Freud, "it is surely of the essence of an emotion that we should be aware of it, i.e. that it should become known to consciousness. Thus, the possibility of the attribute of unconsciousness would be completely excluded as far as emotions, feelings and affects are concerned" (*ibid.*: 179).[8] On the other hand, from his neuroscience perspective, Damasio (1999: 71–79) claims that consciousness is not needed for emotional responses to take place since these are engaged automatically: "we do not learn to wince with pain, we just wince" (*ibid.*: 73). (See also LeDoux, 1998: 54–72.) It is worth noting that, in a social psychology investigation, Poole and Craig (1992) observed that facial expressions of pain remain stable across one's life-span and attempts to mask them do not prevent others from identifying them.

In conclusion, these different approaches to pain contend that, though the invisible, internal character of pain makes it inaccessible to direct observation, its external manifestations (regulatory reactions and pain-induced emotional responses) can be directly observed, thus, turning the private experience into public behaviour. Such observable reactions include, among others, what Hallberg and Carlsson (2000: 34) define as 'overt behavioural expressions', e.g. crying, weeping, and whining, and 'body signals', e.g. facial expressions, touching, and rubbing. Most importantly, people also claim their pain verbally. By means of these verbalisations, they aim at expressing, describing, and qualifying their pain experience. Pain behaviour, therefore, comprises these two observable and hence external accompaniments of the presumed internal state of pain, characterised by Gustafson as 'identifying conditions' (Gustafson, 1979: 156). (See also Fabrega and Tyma, 1976b: 350.)

It is worth noting here that, with respect to emotions in general, from his expressive semantics perspective, Foolen (1997: 19–21) draws an interesting qualitative distinction between the verbal saying and the non-verbal showing of emotions. In the non-verbal, i.e. paralinguistic, way of communication the emotion is

8. Yet, Freud (1915c/1984: 181) argues, in psychoanalytic practice it is observed that repression can succeed "not only in withholding things from consciousness, but also in preventing the development of affect and the setting-off of muscular activity." The term 'unconscious' affects is used for those affects whose development has been inhibited by repression.

expressed *directly*, whereas in a verbal utterance the emotion is *indirectly* communicated since it is first conceptualised and then verbalised, i.e. it is the conceptualisation of the feeling which is communicated. Along the same lines, in their cognitive semantics account, Enfield and Wierzbicka (2002: 6) argue that, being internal, necessarily personal and individualised events, emotions are never communicated directly but rather only descriptions of them in terms of publicly conventionalised signs which are most often linguistic.

2.2.2 What is language for pain?

Verbal avowals and descriptions of pain represent its linguistic dimension, whereby it may be communicated: on the one hand, the sufferer attempts to put his pain into words so that another person might understand it, i.e. he seeks to assign visibility to his otherwise invisible, interior experience, and on the other, the listener tries to 'decode' it. In essence, it is the distinction between the 'private' and 'public' aspect of pain which introduces the relation of language to pain.

For Jackson (1994: 220), "pain, in a sense, is a language", given that it is only through expression that we get aware of the pain of others. Kugelmann (1999: 1668–1669) argues that pain, being invisible, is not independent of the sufferer's persuasive abilities and of its expression through which it gains visibility. "Precisely because it is invisible, does everyone involved seek to reveal it." This leads to the assumption that pain which is not verbally expressed remains private and as such cannot be treated as part of social reality.

Yet, Scarry (1985) has claimed, physical pain is essentially inexpressible, that is, it resists language. According to her, it is the resistance of pain to language that ensures the unsharability of another person's physical pain resulting from its invisibility. What is more, she argues (*ibid.*: 4), "Physical pain does not simply resist language but actively destroys it, bringing about an immediate reversion to a state anterior to language, to the sounds and cries a human being makes before language is learned." An association of pain language with cries, groans, and other pre-language primitive reactions is also made by Wittgenstein in his philosophical 'private language' argument, as we shall see below. However, Scarry (*ibid.*: 13) makes a major point, namely, that despite the inexpressibility of pain, "under the pressure of the desire to eliminate pain, an at least fragmentary means of verbalization is available both to those who are themselves in pain and to those who wish to speak on behalf of others."

"There is no pain [...] without pain behavior", Wittgenstein suggests (1953/1989: 97, § 281). Goldstein (2000: 92) goes as far as to suggest that Wittgenstein essentially proposes that a person is in pain when his behaviour and environment are appropriate, regardless of what sensation, if any, he feels. On the other hand, Wittgenstein also points out that someone may have pain without showing it. Hence, we should not misinterpret his statement quoted above as an implication that there exists no pain when the painful sensation is not verbalised, which would mean that pain is no more than the words used to report the experience (see also Merskey, 1994: S72). Moreover, we should not disregard that there are cases of language impairment (e.g. as a result of advanced age, dementia, illness, etc.) where verbal expression is restricted or impossible. In addition, we should not assume that there is no suffering when patients are silent, given that their silence may sometimes be induced by cultural and spiritual beliefs, as Waddie (1996: 871), from the perspective of advanced nursing science professionals, points out.

2.2.2.1 *Wittgenstein's 'private language argument' and pain*

Wittgenstein's understanding of pain and his philosophical concept of 'private language' will provide us with insights into the interrelation of pain and language. Thus, as regards inner sensations and private experience in general, he claims that the essential thing is that nobody knows whether other people also have the same exemplar as their own or something else. In particular, for Wittgenstein pain is private in the sense that "only I can know whether I am really in pain; another person can only surmise it" (1953/1989: 89, § 246). Moreover, as it is difficult to identify "my pains", it follows that we cannot think of a situation where another person would "have my pains". Similarly, "I can only *believe* that someone else is in pain, but I *know* it if I am" (*ibid.*: 102, § 303). Therefore, according to Wittgenstein, if I say of someone that "he has tooth-ache" I presume that he has what I have when I have tooth-ache. That is, being subjective, pain can only indirectly be identified: each individual experiences his own pain and cannot directly tap the experience of another person (see also Merskey, 1994: S72).

The following question is crucial in any treatment of the language of sensations: how do people relate sensations, which are inner, private experiences, to sensation names, which have intersubjective meaning? Is there something about the way sensations are identified and individuated that allows the words we use as their names to function intersubjectively? How can public language represent a sensation, which is only privately experienced within the individual's body?

Sensations not being public, it cannot be assumed that sensation names are learned ostensively like the words that name public, i.e. observable, objects that people can point to (see Goldstein, 2000: 89). To answer this question, Wittgenstein considers two possibilities, namely, that people might name sensations, either through direct, introspective acquaintance with their own inner experiences, or by attaching a word to the sensation's outward signs. The consideration of these two possibilities is presented in his famous 'private language argument' whereby he rejects the first interpretation and argues in favour of the second one.

Thus, Wittgenstein introduces the concept of a private language in which a person could verbally express his inner experiences (either by speech or writing) for his own private use. Therefore, such a language would be private in two senses: it would refer to only that person's immediate sensations and it would also be private in the sense of being understood only by him. "And sounds which no one else understands but which I '*appear to understand*' might be called a 'private language'" (Wittgenstein, 1953/1989: 94, § 269). Wittgenstein suggests that this private language would consist of words that a person would arbitrarily and directly associate with his own sensations, whose intrinsic character he would be the only one to know.

To render his philosophical concept more familiar, he invites us to imagine that someone experiences a particular sensation and decides to use 'S' as a sensation name to refer to it whenever it occurs thereafter. Wittgenstein sees two fundamental weaknesses in this naming process, however. Not only would such a word be understood exclusively by the person himself, but, most importantly, he would lack any criterion of correctness, since he would be unable to retrieve the initial sensation he had when he first introduced 'S' as a sensation name. Therefore, no definition of the sign 'S' could be formulated; only an ostensive definition to the person himself could inwardly be provided, which, however, could not be assessed for its correctness. Wittgenstein uses a very vivid metaphor to support his argument. He argues that if a person gives himself a private definition of a word it is as if his right hand has given his left hand money: we cannot really see this as a gift.

The question, therefore, remains as to how words are made to refer to sensations, i.e. how the connection between the name and a sensation is established, which is another way of asking how human beings learn the meaning of sensation names, e.g. of the word 'pain'. Having considered the possibility that people acquire such knowledge through the direct, introspective acquaintance involved in a 'private' language, Wittgenstein (*ibid.*: 89, § 244) turns to the second possibility and suggests:

> Words are connected with the primitive, the natural, expressions of the sensation and used in their place. A child has hurt himself and he cries; and then adults talk to him and teach him exclamations and, later, sentences. They teach the child new pain-behaviour.

To stress the role of outward signs in teaching and learning pain words, Wittgenstein argues that groaning, grimacing and other natural pain manifestations are a necessary condition of teaching a child the use of 'tooth-ache', for example, as the name of a personal experience. Thus, outward signs to which we pin the use of sensation names are the means whereby we are able to establish the intersubjective reference of verbal expressions of the pain sensation. Wittgenstein essentially endorses the view that a sensation name is intersubjective and, therefore, can be established and learned, only if the sensation is accompanied by concurrent outward signs which he assumes to be public, in the sense that they might be understood by someone else. (For an interpretation of Wittgenstein's argument as well as a different proposal concerning the way we learn sensation names in terms of the intersubjective properties of mental states, see Goldstein, 2000.)[9] It follows, therefore, that the language that describes my sensations cannot be 'private'. Conclusively, no private language could be used in a game of naming sensations as part of a public behaviour, namely the expression of pain. Only our ordinary language can serve the purpose of publicly expressing and legitimising pain.[10] It is through the medium of speech that a person communicates his pain, after being taught to connect the word 'pain' with his private experience in much the same way as he associates the name of a colour with a particular, private impression of the colour in him.

In Kripke's (1982: 100) understanding, for Wittgenstein, "outward criteria for an inner process are circumstances, observable in the behaviour of an individual, which, when present, would lead others to agree with his avowals." Kripke (*ibid.*:

9. Goldstein (2000: 91-92) argues that for Wittgenstein "outward signs give conditions necessary and sufficient for the correct use of psychological words." Therefore, 'the intersubjectivity=outward signs postulate' plays a central role in his private language argument. Goldstein rejects the two possible ways considered by Wittgenstein concerning how people may name sensations, i.e. (a) direct introspective acquaintance and (b) outward signs. He proposes a third method whereby sensation names are learnable non-ostensively, in terms of intersubjective formal properties by which we identify and individuate mental states. Thus, according to him, a sensation has some qualitative character or *quale* which is identified by abstract, formal properties. It is in terms of these specifiable properties that a *quale* is analysable. In particular, with regard to pain, he distinguishes between first-order and second-order properties and argues that, like every unpleasant sensation, pain has a specific qualitative character (quale) having the abstract, formal, second-order property of being intrinsically bad. This second-order property supervenes on pain's first-order properties (e.g. spatiotemporal features, causes and effects) which, however, are not defining properties of pain and are learnable only through experience. For Goldstein, when a person knows *what the word 'pain' means* he knows something about *what pain is* and, therefore, something about its second-order property of being intrinsically bad, i.e. *how pain feels*. He points out, however, that knowing specific, defining, first-order properties of particular pains "is not part of knowing what pain means though may be part of knowing what pain is." "Using words that name sensations by formal properties we refer to events that have first-order properties whose character can be known only through direct acquaintance" (*ibid.*: 101). Goldstein's main thesis is that the 'inward process' he proposes, whereby a person's knowledge of sensation names is acquired in terms of formal properties, "does not stand in need of outward criteria" (*ibid.*: 102). Conclusively, he claims that it is formal criteria which structure how we talk about both the public and physical and the private and mental.

10. The idea that pain is validated through language is also to be found in Engel (1950), where it is suggested that verbal declaration is what marks the transition from private to public pain. Therefore, when expressed verbally, pain becomes part of a social relationship.

102–103) further remarks that Wittgenstein's account often seems to be misinterpreted to the effect that it is assumed that for every kind of sensation there is a corresponding natural expression, i.e. an outward criterion. Consequently, to each avowal of the type "I have a sensation *S*" there must also be an outward criterion associated with *S* and it is by virtue of it that others may recognise the presence or absence of *S*. However, he argues that it seems likely that such a view is *empirically* false and provides the following justification: "It seems to me that we have sensations or sensation *qualia* that we can perfectly well identify but that have no 'natural' external manifestations; an observer cannot tell in any way whether an individual has them unless that individual avows them."

In fact, Wittgenstein further elaborates his argument by asking on what criteria besides external manifestation we can judge that a person is experiencing or has experienced a sensation. His answer to this question reveals the fundamental difference between undergoing an experience and simply observing another person undergoing one. That is, he suggests that, with respect to someone else, the only criteria I can rely on are outward signs, whereas for myself I unquestionably know whether I have an experience.

There is, however, some contradiction involved in the linguistic manifestation of pain: it relates inner sensations and emotions that are strictly private, on the one hand, to linguistic expressions which are assumed to be understood by all the members of a linguistic society, on the other (see Jones, 1975/1997). How is this link effected? What is the basis of this delicate and obscure relationship? The most plausible interpretation is expressed in the assumption that in pain, as in other subjective conditions, there are "common phenomena which seem to be the same from person to person or case to case" (Merskey, 1994: S72). That is, despite its private, subjective, and invisible nature, pain constitutes a common domain of human experience.

Returning to Wittgenstein, if we interpret and extend his discussion of the word 'red' as a sensation name, we will understand that he is essentially addressing the same crucial question: is it that words for sensations mean something known to everyone and in addition, for each person, they also mean – or rather refer to – something known only to him? Thus, he suggests, though I use the word 'toothache' in a game I play with other people, i.e. a public one, the word also has a private meaning to me. He then wonders how we can be certain that we all attach the same meaning to the word 'pain', since everyone knows what it means only from his own experience and suggests (Wittgenstein, 1953/1989: 100, § 295):

> Suppose everyone does say about himself that he knows what pain is only from his own pain. – Not that people really say that, or are even prepared to say it. But *if* everybody said it – it might be a kind of exclamation. And even if it gives no in-

> formation, still it is a picture, and why should we not want to call up such a picture? Imagine an allegorical painting take the place of those words.

2.2.2.2 *The function of pain language: Expressive and/or descriptive?*

The issue of the basic role of pain language, i.e. its function as an expressive and/or descriptive device, is raised by Wittgenstein's view that individuals, as children, are taught, somewhat artificially, to use particular words as labels for subjective painful experiences, so as to replace crying and other primitive, natural, expressions.

Thus, for him "the verbal expression of pain replaces crying and does not describe it" (*ibid.*: 89, § 244), essentially forming part of the pain experience itself. For example, a child is taught to use the words "I have a tooth-ache" to replace its moans.[11] Interpreting this view, Kripke (1982: 135) argues that an avowal of pain – which is a more sophisticated pain behaviour, a substitute for the primitive non-verbal expression of pain – need not be based on any special application of criteria any more than a cry is and adds that "in the most primitive case it *escapes* from the speaker." Moreover, we may infer from a point Wittgenstein (1953/1989: 91, § 256) makes later in his discussion that, in the absence of natural expressions, language would not be used to replace them and, therefore, would not have an expressive function but, rather, linguistic forms would be used simply to refer to sensations and produce descriptions. Most importantly, referring to particular linguistic manifestations of inner experiences and relating "I am in pain" with "I am afraid", he poses the crucial question: should they be understood as (a) descriptions of a state of mind or (b) cries of complaint which are more primitive than any description and, therefore, do not qualify as descriptions? Thus, in the following famous quotes (*ibid.*: 189) he touches upon the dual function of pain avowals:

> A cry is not a description. But there are transitions. And the words "I am afraid" may approximate more, or less, to being a cry. They may come quite close to this and also be *far* removed from it.
> We surely do not always say someone is *complaining*, because he says he is in pain. So the words "I am in pain" may be a cry of complaint, and may be something else.

11. Departing from Wittgenstein's philosophical speculation and moving to actual research on a related issue, namely, the acquisition of emotion language by two-year-old infants, I am tempted to quote the results of research carried out by Bloom (1993a) and (1993b) as reported in Foolen (1997: 19–20): "words did not replace affect expression in the period of word learning, and speech was not something these children did instead of expressing emotion. Rather, they were beginning to learn language as a new system of expression for the contents and their beliefs and desires while they continued to express their feelings about these contents through displays of affect" (Bloom, 1993b: 104).

Elaborating the main claims extractable from these passages, Gustafson (1979: 153–155) argues that the grammatical point made about 'pain' is that it is not primarily and intrinsically a descriptive term of felt quality. That is, pains are not merely ostensively identifiable since they can be "identified, referred to, speculated about, compared and contrasted in the absence of felt *qualia*." In addition, Gustafson suggests, Wittgenstein essentially claims that, depending on the context of their occurrence, avowals of pain can be either self-descriptions or primitive expressive reactions. In other words, Wittgenstein draws an important distinction between the primary, basic role of avowals of pain which he describes as 'manifestations', 'expressions', 'natural cries' etc., on the one hand, and derived, more sophisticated uses of verbal pain utterances, on the other. The dual function of pain language is very insightfully captured in Kenny's (1973) interpretation (as reported in Gustafson, 1979: 154), according to which

> "I am in pain" is a manifestation of pain – *via* a complaint (or cry) – or is a manifestation of pain in a linguistic mode derived from and dependent upon the function in our lives of cries, manifestations, responses to injury, and so on. The linguistic expression *can* function as a description, however.

Thus, we see that the linguistic manifestation of pain is understood primarily as an expression of this sensation, or as also potentially entailing a description. What is more, the distinction between expression and description cannot always be sharply drawn, since it allows for 'transitions' between linguistic configurations approximating more to functioning as either a cry or a description. Emphasis is also given to the role of the context in interpreting our pain avowals as expressive or descriptive utterances, though quite often the expressive function of spontaneous pain verbalisations serves others as a description of our painful sensations. In a related passage Wittgenstein (1953/1989: 96–97, § 280) metaphorically relates our impression of a colour, e.g. red, with the picture that someone would draw to show how he imagined a theatre scene. He suggests that this picture would have a double function, i.e. it would inform others, since, like words, pictures are informative, but it would also be a subjective representation of the scene "in a sense in which the picture cannot mean this to others." If we extend the view essentially expressed here to the role of verbal manifestations of pain, we may assume that it highlights their double function: by providing descriptive accounts, they may inform others and, for the sufferer, they are representations reflecting his own experience, i.e. expressions rather than descriptions. Thus, a description is other-oriented and informative, whereas an expression is self-oriented.

In Lascaratou and Hatzidaki (2002: 71, 56) it was proposed that these functions could be graphically represented in terms of a "primitive reaction – linguistic manifestation (expression and/or description)" integrating continuum which would cover "manifestations of pain ranging from the primitive cry – through automatic and impulsive pain avowals – to descriptive, reportive and objectifying linguistic configurations." Moreover, in that first taxonomy of Greek lexico-phraseological forms and constructions of pain it was claimed that, due to their predominantly intransitive personal character, *ponao* 'I hurt' / 'I'm hurting' pain avowals profile pain as a holistic experience, and thus relate to the more expressive side of the spectrum, often approximating to the primitive cry. On the other hand, in Lascaratou and Marmaridou (2005) it is argued that the opposite pole of the continuum can be seen as featuring *ponos* 'pain' nominal constructions, which are systematically motivated by conceptual metaphors, lending themselves to the objectification of pain, hence enabling the sufferer to formulate explicit descriptions of the experience. Additional empirical evidence in support of the suggested schematic representation of the linguistic manifestation of pain as expression – transition – description will be provided in my subsequent data analysis. What is more, in the light of Foolen's (1997) study of the expressive function of language (which will be presented in more detail in section 6.2) and the distinction he draws between direct and indirect communication of emotions, in particular, I shall attempt to further refine my interpretation of the expressive vs. descriptive function of pain language.

According to Foolen's (1997) proposed analysis of the communication of cognitive and emotional content, while verbal utterances can serve the purpose of *directly* communicating ideas (cognition), they can only *indirectly* communicate emotions (affect), the direct communication channel of the latter being non-verbal utterances, i.e. paralinguistic means. Thus, he argues that emotion can be externalised in two qualitatively different ways: through the direct, paralinguistic, channel, namely non-verbal showing, and in the indirect way, through verbal saying, whereby, he suggests, the emotion is first conceptualised and then verbalised. Foolen then addresses a crucial question: is there a direct linguistic expression of emotions, i.e. one leading directly from emotion to verbal utterance, without the intermediary step of conceptualisation?

Extending Foolen's question about a potential direct verbal mode of expressing emotion to the communication of pain, I shall venture to map my analysis of the linguistic dimension of pain in Greek onto his account of the communication of emotion: in my proposed representation, the (proto)typical expressive function is assigned to the direct non-verbal communication of pain (i.e. automatic pain reactions, e.g. cries / groans / screams), while the descriptive function is assigned to indirectly (*via* cognition) externalised pain verbalisations. As an attempt to provide an answer to his question, I shall propose that the linguistic manifestation of pain does *not always* constitute an *indirect* channel of communication, but rather there are also cases of *directly* communicated verbal utterances, namely, instances of intransitive first-person *ponao* 'I hurt' / 'I'm hurting' or impersonal third-person *ponai* 'it hurts' / 'it's hurting' pain avowals.

2.2.2.3 *How is pain transformed into language?*

Having speculated on the private and public aspects of pain and the role of its linguistic dimension in expressing and describing it, i.e. rendering it public, the following question addressed by Fabrega and Tyma (1976: 353) inevitably emerges and calls for an answer: "How and on what basis is pain, a perceptual experience, given meaning and significance by means of language?" How do the linguistic symbols of pain (words, phrases), which are arbitrarily and conventionally linked to the pain experience, acquire the meaning attributed to them?

The view put forward by Halliday (1998: 23–24) about the significance of lexico-grammar in construing semantically our experiential domains of everyday life in general and pain in particular, i.e. in understanding the world, provides an answer to this question from a functional linguistic perspective. However, Halliday points out, the lexico-grammatical categories used should not be *ad hoc* but should be part of a general theory-based description of language:

> If we try to reflect casually on the language used to construe such everyday domains, we may come up with a few lexical items – single words, and perhaps a common phrase or two. But we will not be able to comprehend how the real work of making meaning is done unless we probe more deeply, into the vaults of the grammar. Grammar is the source of energy, the semogenic powerhouse of language. It is in grammar that our world takes shape.

Halliday's (1998) account of English pain expressions within the broader framework of Functional Grammar (Halliday, 1985/1994) having served as the theoretical ground of this long-term study, one of the basic assumptions underlying this investigation has been that "the encoding of pain in language does not simply involve the attachment of words as labels to painful sensations, but most importantly the construal of this domain of unpleasant experience in terms of structural configurations" (Lascaratou and Hatzidaki, 2002: 56).[12] Hence, in studying the lexico-grammar of pain and, thus, revealing how the various complex aspects of this domain of human experience are construed in language, I aim at attempting

12. The complexity of this issue is vividly brought out in an interesting comment made by Melzack and Torgerson (1971: 53-54) on the multitude of pain words and the vastness of the pain experience: they point out that, on the one hand, the existence of so many words to describe pain shows that the word 'pain' is a label representing a myriad of different experiences, but, on the other hand, our linguistic labels are restricted and narrow symbolic verbal categories compared to our experiences.

to provide an answer to the central question motivating this investigation, i.e. "what is pain for language?".

It is worth noting that, seen from a purely philosophical rather than linguistic perspective, the fundamental role of grammar in the process of verbalising pain is stressed in Wittgenstein's (1953/1989: 92, § 257) oft-quoted very insightful remark that even the mere act of naming (pain) presupposes the existence of grammar, which, by means of the stage-setting it creates, "shews the post where the new word is stationed." Yet, we should be careful not to misinterpret Wittgenstein's use of the term *grammar* as strictly referring to concrete grammatical features as these are understood in a clearly linguistic approach, e.g. Halliday's functional approach. Rather, Wittgenstein uses *grammar* as a philosophical concept whereby the conceptualisation of our world of experience through language is understood (See Wittgenstein, 1969/1974). Hence, for him "essence is expressed by grammar" and "grammar tells us what kind of object something is" (Wittgenstein, 1953/1989: 116, § 371 and § 373).

Assuming with Gustafson (1979: 151–152) that the term 'object' is not used here to refer strictly to object-entities, I shall adopt his alternative broader interpretation of Wittgenstein's view expressed in this philosophical dictum. More specifically, it seems plausible to infer that 'object' is used in a broad sense as a cover term to refer to processes, i.e. states and activities, as well as objects. Therefore, I understand this statement as capturing the role played by Wittgenstein's philosophical concept of grammar in conceptualising our experience in general. That Wittgenstein sees a close relation between concepts and his understanding of grammar is further revealed in his remark that we learn the concept 'pain' when we learn language.

2.2.3 What is pain for language?

In my attempt to answer this question with respect to Greek, I am essentially endorsing Gustafson's (1979: 151–152) claim that, quite often in inquiry, we start with an initial idea of the kind of thing something is (*what* kind) which arises from

> our more or less explicit account of the grammar of the words, the language of and about, the thing in question. Inquiry is then often directed to the question *which* kind this kind is; for instance, given that it is, grammatically, a process, we then ask which kind of process is it?

Interestingly, the following theoretical issues – both '*what* kind' and '*which* kind' questions, i.e. referring to two different levels of specificity – addressed by M.A.K. Halliday (1998: 11) and expressed in clearly functional linguistic terms, which have served as my point of departure in investigating how pain is represented in the Greek language, could be seen as echoing Wittgenstein's philosophical claim that grammar tells us what kind of object something is:

> What type of element is 'pain'? Is it process, participant, or circumstance? Is it a quality of something? If participant, or quality, is it construed circumstantially? Does it involve the relationship between one process configuration and another? And, in terms of any of these elements, is it simple or complex? And is it consistently construed in one way, or does it vary among different modes of construal? In other words, where does pain fit in to the configuration of everyday experience?

By providing answers to the questions he poses with respect to English and organising the most typical pain expressions into a working paradigm within the framework of Functional Grammar, Halliday (1998) offers us the necessary theoretical framework for the investigation of the construal of pain as process, participant, quality or circumstance in Greek (see Chapter 4). Conclusively, extending Halliday's analysis to the pain configurations observed in my Greek doctor-patient data, I shall venture to portray how pain is profiled by the Greek language, which should, ultimately, contribute to an understanding of how pain is perceived by the sufferer.

CHAPTER 3

Corpus design and data collection

This research project is founded on one of the fundamental assumptions underlying corpus linguistics, namely, that intuition about language cannot reliably and objectively detect or predict patterns of usage in the absence of factual evidence emerging from natural language data: one's intuitions should be guided by and supplemented with evidence compiled objectively from a computerised corpus of naturally-occurring language data rather than from elicited or invented language. (See Sinclair, 1991: 4; Deignan, 1999a: 178; Deignan, 1999b: 20; and Deignan, 2005b: 27, 88.) In particular, with respect to the investigation of the linguistic aspect of pain, it is my belief that it could not possibly be based on the researcher's intuitions and his or her personal observations only, given that pain is not experienced in a single way by different people, but rather it is a unique experience for each individual, due to its subjective, complex, and multi-faceted nature. In other words, the linguistic dimension of pain being a reflection of the diversity and complexity of this universal, yet very private, domain of everyday life, one would not be able to gain insights into how pain is perceived and experienced unless one looked into the language spontaneously used by a considerable number of pain suffering individuals. This view essentially coincides with Halliday's (1998: 7) suggestion that "for 'pain' in the grammar of daily life one would need to use a corpus of spontaneous spoken language."[1]

Moreover, the corpus of this study was designed within the constraints involved in the understanding of pain in terms of its currently accepted definition recommended by the International Association for the Study of Pain (IASP), namely, that pain is "an unpleasant sensory and emotional experience associated with actual or potential tissue damage, or described in terms of such damage." Since the painful experience is associated with or described in terms of (actual or potential) tissue damage, it follows that the IASP definition adopted in this study assigns a central role to such damage. Assuming the fundamental role of physical or other causes experienced as physical ones emerging from the IASP definition, it

1. For a presentation of explicit discussions of the methodological issues and techniques used in corpus-based work, with a primary emphasis on the interesting investigations of language use possible through this approach, see Biber, Conrad and Reppen (1998).

was decided not to include linguistic expressions used in everyday encounters as a means of denoting mere psychological discomfort but instead to restrict the data collection to utterances produced in a health care context, where, by definition, physical pain is exposed (i.e. described or expressed) or even produced.[2] These considerations motivated my decision to proceed with the collection of a corpus of naturally-occurring dialogues between pain-suffering patients and health care professionals (doctors, physiotherapists and psychologists).[3] Hence, a so-called 'bottom-up' approach was selected. (For a discussion of the advantages of adopting a bottom-up approach in the analysis of the metaphorical conceptualisation of pain and the benefits of merging this type of approach to the 'top-down' one followed by cognitive scholars, see Chapter 8, section 8.1.)

The collected material amounts to 69,996 words (tokens) and consists of 131 different spontaneous dialogues recorded between January 2000 and October 2001. These were naturally produced by 131 different patients and 8 medical professionals from 5 hospitals and practices in Athens who agreed to participate in the study. The majority of the data, i.e. 60.22%, (42,149 words) derives from musculoskeletal-related medical discourse; 15.68% (10,975 words), recorded in the pain management clinic of a general hospital, represents dialogues with patients suffering from a variety of pathological problems (e.g. urine infection, pain after a kidney operation, oro-facial pain, migraine, etc.) as well as musculoskeletal ones; the remaining 24.10%, i.e. almost one fourth of the material (16,872 words), is covered by conversations with cancer patients in the pain management clinic of a cancer

2. The material of this study does not include utterances used to express psychological discomfort unrelated to or not described in terms of physical causes, e.g. *me ponai na se vlepo na ise toso apelpizmeni* 'it hurts me to see you being so desperate', *ponao otan katalaveno oti δen me njazese* 'I hurt / I feel pain when I realise that you don't care for me.'

3. For a comparison of three of the most commonly used approaches to the analysis of data from doctor-patient interaction, see Thomas and Wilson (1996).

hospital.[4] Recordings were transcribed orthographically, whilst no prosodic or other annotation was added.

A combined qualitative and quantitative methodology, drawing on tools widely used for corpus analysis was applied: the first step was to read the corpus end-to-end in search of potential clues to patterns; these were then used as starting points for the subsequent automated searches in the electronic corpus. (See Cameron and Deignan, 2003.) On the basis of automatically extracted concordances and statistical data, patterns and their frequencies were identified using the Wordsmith Tools 3.0 corpus processing software, while manual coding was applied to characterize their nature and function.

The relatively small size of the corpus – compared to the usual size of general corpora – is largely due to the unexpected reluctance to cooperate expressed, unfortunately, by the majority of health professionals: in most cases, the medical personnel displayed a negative attitude, refusing to have their sessions recorded, despite my explicit assurance that confidentiality and anonymity rules would be observed. Since the corpus of this study was from the start not intended as a general corpus, i.e. one which attempts to represent a language as a whole, its size is counterbalanced by its very specialised nature: it is a coherent, intensively studied, electronic corpus of dialogues extracted from the specific context of medical discourse with *ponao* verb patterns and *ponos* nominal constructions in focus. (For the value of specialised small corpora "delimited by a register, discourse domain, or subject-matter", see de Beaugrande, 2001: 23.)

It should be noted that a number of obstacles have made it practically impossible to draw a random sample of conversations on the basis of a pre-established demographic design (Crowdy, 1993). The first concerns the unexpected unwillingness to cooperate on the part of the majority of medical professionals mentioned

4. One might consider the possibility that the focus on musculoskeletal pain data (which was not originally intended but rather eventually occurred as a result of some physicians' reluctance to assist me with the data collection) may have constrained the observed linguistic manifestations of pain to some unknown extent (such as the variety and frequency of collected lexicogrammatical items and structures as well as the sets of metaphors). In that respect, it would be challenging to compare the findings of this project with a future study focusing on the linguistic aspect of pain related to other systems of the human body, such as the neurological system, or specific organs, e.g. headaches and migraines. In addition, from the exploration of the dialogues with cancer-patients, I suspect that a systematic study of pain data from terminal diseases might show the prevalence of specific aspects of the linguistic dimension of pain, e.g. an extensive use of metaphors to describe the mixture of physical pain and despair experienced in fatal conditions and the paralysing / confining effect that such pain may often produce. On the other hand, a small sample of labour pain data that I have collected seems to indicate that the language used is very strongly constrained by the particular unique context of situation where physical pain is mixed with the anticipation of a very happy event.

above. The second difficulty is a consequence of the actual routine conditions under which doctor-patient sessions are regularly conducted: it is practically impossible for a health professional to select his patients according to demographic criteria. To counteract these negative effects and achieve the highest possible degree of representativeness, care was taken to ensure that as many participants as possible were included, and thus avoid the skewing normally caused by low speaker variation (see Biber, 1993; Gibbon, Moore and Winski, 1998).

The corpus includes pain language observed in two, often interrelated, types of authentic communicative situations, namely, utterances produced while patients are exposing their painful experiences, e.g. in a pain management clinic or in the course of a medical consultation, but also spontaneous verbal reactions to the infliction of pain at the time of the recording, e.g. during a physiotherapy session. It was my assumption that such face-to-face conversations should be abundant in pain language and my expectation that a wide range of diverse pain utterances could, therefore, be collected that motivated the selection of these text types. My expectation was further supported by Halliday's remark that, despite its very short length, the medical consultation dialogue he analysed contained "a remarkable amount of variation within a small number of instances" and that in itself it was "a critical feature of the way that pain comes to be construed" (*ibid.*: 9). My initial assumption about the usefulness and direct relevance of such data for my linguistic investigation was strongly confirmed by a *post hoc* observation concerning the frequency of two word forms, which constitute fundamental tools for the communication of pain in Greek. More specifically, in the corpus, on the one hand, the verbal form *ponai* 'it hurts' / 'it's hurting' is not only the most frequent verb after the delexical form *ine* 'is' / 'are', but it is also the most frequent lexical word overall, and, on the other, the form *ponos* 'pain' is by far the most frequent noun. (For the use of such data-driven or *internal* criteria for the evaluation of corpus structure, see Sinclair, 1994 and Hatzidaki, 1999.)

The medical experts were contacted on a personal basis and the nature and goal of the project were explained to them. Those who agreed to participate were given the necessary equipment in order to tape-record their interaction with pain suffering patients. All patients who participated were aware of the recording process and had given their consent in advance, i.e. all recordings were *visible* (Gibbon, Moore and Winski, 1998). Clandestine recording was ruled out as unethical (Holmes, 1996). However, the real aim of the recording procedure, i.e. the collection of data for linguistic analysis, was not revealed to the patients, as the health care professionals were advised against disclosing it and were given instructions to tell the patients that the purposes of the recording were entirely medical, e.g. keeping full records of each case.

This was a distracting technique (cf. Edwards and Pearce, 1994) applied in order to minimise the potential distorting effect of two variables on the linguistic authenticity of the non-surreptitiously collected material, namely, the variable of *good subject tendency* and that of *evaluation apprehension* (McBurney, 1994: 29). In particular, with respect to the first variable, it has been observed that subjects tend "to act according to what they think the [researcher] wants," while, according to the second one, they tend to "alter their behaviour in order to appear as socially desirable as possible." On the other hand, it is my belief that the subjective and emotional aspect of the pain experience had an increasing effect on the genuineness and naturalness of the language produced, despite the patients' awareness of the session being recorded. (For the role of emotional involvement as a factor triggering unattended forms of speech even in the course of a recording process, see Gibbon, Moore and Winski, 1998: 105.)

CHAPTER 4

Mode of analysis

4.1 Introduction

In order to be able to show how pain is transformed into meaning by grammar, it is not sufficient to simply analyse the language of this domain of human experience in lexico-grammatical terms and come up with an inventory of lexico-phraseological forms and syntactic structures. It is a necessary condition that our analysis be based on a theoretical model, i.e. categories which "are not *ad hoc* but are part of a general theory-based description of the language" (Halliday, 1998: 23).

It is precisely to meet this necessary condition that I am adopting as my theoretical framework Halliday's (1998) functional account of English pain expressions. This approach lends itself to being used as a theoretical basis for the study of the construal of pain by languages other than English by virtue of its organisation into a pre-systemic form within the more general framework of Functional Grammar. By displaying and organising the most representative English expressions of pain into a working paradigm from the standpoint of transitivity, Halliday is able to compare and contrast them systematically in terms of their grammatical features. Thus, Halliday provides us with a theoretical ground that may be extended so as to serve as the necessary basis required in a functional analysis of the linguistic dimension of pain in Greek.

In the following section, I shall briefly sketch those aspects of Halliday's (1985/1994) Functional Grammar that will enable me to create the necessary stage setting for the presentation and interpretation of my data along the lines of his paradigm of pain expressions. In particular, I shall summarise the basic points of his understanding of the 'experiential' function of the clause, i.e. "its guise as a way of representing patterns of experience" (*ibid.*: 106), by virtue of the general principle embodied by the clause, i.e. that reality is made up of PROCESSES or 'goings-on', such as happening, doing, sensing, meaning, and being and becoming.[1]

1. The examples used in this chapter belong to Halliday (1985/1994).

4.2 Halliday's process types in modelling experience

Transitivity is the grammatical system whereby the world of experience is construed into a manageable set of process types. The grammar distinguishes rather clearly between our outer experience, the processes of the external world, and our inner experience, the processes of consciousness, and sets up the grammatical categories of material processes and mental processes, respectively. The grammar also recognises relational processes, i.e. those of classifying and identifying. Material, mental and relational are the three main types of process in the English transitivity system, at the boundaries of which three more process types are located, namely, behavioural, verbal, and existential processes. For Halliday, there is no priority of one type of process over another, which he shows by ordering them in a continuum forming a circle rather than a line. Using a visual metaphor on the analogy of colour, he suggests that

> the grammar construes experience like a colour chart, with red, blue and yellow as primary colours and purple, green and orange along the borders; not like a physical spectrum, with red at one end and violet at the other (Halliday, 1985/1994: 107).

A process consists of three components: (i) the process itself, (ii) participants in the process, and (iii) optionally, circumstances associated with the process. It is important to understand that these three concepts, namely, process, participant, and circumstance are semantic categories "which explain in the most general way how phenomena of the real world are represented as linguistic structure" (*ibid.*: 109). It is this tripartite interpretation of processes that underlies the grammatical distinction of words into lexical classes, i.e. verbs, nouns, etc., "a pattern that in some way or other is probably universal among human languages" (*ibid.*: 108). Hence, in Halliday's understanding, the process is typically realised by the verbal group of the clause, participants are realised by nominal groups, while circumstances are realised by adverbial groups or prepositional phrases. (For a cognitive account of semantic structure and the notional basis of fundamental grammatical categories such as noun, verb, adjective, and adverb, see Langacker, 1987.[2] See also

2. Within the framework of cognitive grammar, Langacker (1987: 182, 189, 244, 491, 494) argues that basic grammatical categories such as noun, verb, adjective, and adverb can be defined semantically. Thus for example, according to him, a noun can be said to designate a thing, and similarly a verb designates a process, or in more technical terms, a noun is definable as a symbolic structure whose semantic pole profiles a thing, while a verb can be defined as a symbolic expression whose semantic pole designates a process. Moreover, he suggests that a process "must have the profile of a relation throughout its temporal extension" (*ibid.*: 247).

Wierzbicka, 1988 for an account of nouns, adjectives and verbs within her proposed framework of 'grammatical semantics'.[3])

MATERIAL processes are processes of 'doing' which express the notion that some entity 'does' something – which may be done 'to' some other entity. In such processes there are two particular participants: an obligatory ACTOR, which is the 'logical Subject' of older terminology, and means the doer of the deed (e.g. *the mouse ran up the clock*), and optionally also a GOAL. Thus, intransitive clauses comprise only an Actor, while transitive clauses comprise both an Actor and a Goal. The Goal function is best defined as the one which the process is 'directed at' or 'extended to' (e.g. *the lion caught the tourist*), though the term PATIENT has also been used, meaning one that 'suffers' or 'undergoes' the process. It is the concept of extension which is in fact embodied in the classical terminology of 'transitive' and 'intransitive', from which the term 'transitivity' is derived.[4]

There are, however, clauses for which, unlike material process clauses, the Actor-Goal trail should be abandoned. These are clauses of feeling, thinking and perceiving, which can be grouped together under the general heading of MENTAL PROCESSES. Thus, the principal sub-types of mental process are PERCEPTION (seeing, hearing etc.), AFFECTION (liking, fearing etc.) and COGNITION (thinking, knowing, understanding etc.). Of the two participants in a mental process, the SENSER, i.e. the being that is feeling, thinking or seeing, is always human or 'endowed with consciousness'. The other main participant, the PHENOMENON, i.e. that which is 'sensed' – felt, thought or seen – may be a 'thing' or a 'fact'. In addition to these distinctive features of their participants, these clauses are grammatically distinct from material process clauses with regard to three more criteria:

1. In mental processes, which in general are not clearly bounded in time, the unmarked present tense is the SIMPLE PRESENT. On the other hand, in material processes, which typically have clear beginnings and endings, the unmarked tense is the PRESENT IN PRESENT (Halliday's term for PRESENT CONTINUOUS), as it is more focused in time. Though both tenses are used with

3. Wierzbicka (1988: 8) argues that the meaning of a sentence is determined and conveyed jointly by the meaning of its words and of its grammatical devices and that drawing any line between the two would inevitably be arbitrary: there are "only lexical and grammatical MEANS of conveying meaning." She claims that, in addition to the intermediary status of 'function words' (e.g. conjunctions, prepositions, etc.), the grammatical status of 'full words' (e.g. nouns, verbs, and adjectives) plays an equally important role. "The very fact that a word is a noun, or an adjective, or a verb, determines some aspects of its meaning", she maintains.

4. If there is a Goal of the process, as well as an Actor, the representation may come in either of two forms: either active, *the lion caught the tourist*, or passive, *the tourist was caught by the lion*.

both types of process, the other one is the marked option in each case, carrying a special interpretation.

2. Mental processes can be realised with the Subject functioning as either the Senser or the Phenomenon, still keeping the clause in the active voice, no parallel to this bidirectionality existing in material process clauses: e.g. *I like it, it pleases me.*
3. Mental processes being processes of feeling, thinking and seeing, are not kinds of 'doing', and, therefore, cannot be probed or substituted by *do*, e.g. **What John did was know the answer.*

One final important difference is that with mental processes there is no 'intransitive' (one participant) / 'transitive' (two participants) distinction: all mental processes potentially involve both a Senser and a Phenomenon. This, however, does not mean that both must always be present in the clause: there can be a Senser and no Phenomenon, e.g. *Jill can't see, Tim knows*, and, conversely, there can be a Phenomenon and no Senser, e.g. *He only does it to annoy.*

RELATIONAL processes could be said to be those of 'being', e.g. *Sarah is wise, Tom is the leader*, but not 'being' in the sense of existing. Rather a relation is being set up between two separate entities, e.g. *x* and *a*. The English system operates with three main types:

1. intensive '*x* is *a*'
2. circumstantial '*x* is at *a*' (where 'is at' stands for 'is at, in, on, for, with, about, along, etc.')
3. possessive '*x* has *a*'

Each of these comes in two distinct modes:

- attributive '*a* is an attribute of *x*'
- identifying '*a* is the identity of *x*'

In particular, with respect to the attributive mode, which will be considered in the analysis of Greek pain constructions, an entity *x* is configured as having some quality *a* ascribed or attributed to it. Structurally, this quality is labelled the ATTRIBUTE, and the entity to which it is ascribed is the CARRIER, i.e. the one that 'carries' the attribute. We can interpret this as '*x* is a member of the class of *a*'.

Besides the three main process types, there are also three subsidiary ones, located at each of the boundaries:

behavioural	sharing characteristics of	material and mental
verbal	sharing characteristics of	mental and relational
existential	sharing characteristics of	relational and material

On the borderline between material and mental are the BEHAVIOURAL processes, that represent outer manifestations of inner workings, the acting out of (typically human) processes of consciousness and physiological states, like breathing, coughing, smiling, dreaming and staring.[5] The participant who is 'behaving', the BEHAVER, is typically a conscious being, like the Senser. The process, however, is grammatically more like one of 'doing', the usual unmarked present tense being present continuous, like the material, e.g. *you're dreaming!* Notably, behavioural processes are almost always middle, i.e. they most typically consist of the Process and only one participant, the Behaver, e.g. *don't breathe!*

On the borderline between mental and relational are the VERBAL processes, i.e. 'symbolic' processes of saying, which cover any kind of symbolic exchange of meaning. Unlike mental processes, verbal processes do not require their typical participant, the SAYER, to be conscious, as long as it is something that communicates a signal, e.g. <u>the notice</u> *tells you to keep quiet*, <u>the light</u> *says stop*, <u>my watch</u> *says it's half past ten.*

On the borderline between the relational and the material are the processes concerned with existence, the EXISTENTIAL, by which phenomena of all kinds that can be construed as a 'thing' (person, object, institution, abstraction, but also any action or event) are simply recognised to 'be' – to exist, or to happen, e.g. *there was a little cat, there seems to be a problem, has there been a phone call?, there isn't enough time, there was another robbery in the street.* Like relational processes, existential clauses typically have the verb *be*. That object or event which is being said to exist is labelled, simply, EXISTENT.

On the borderline between the existential and the material there is a special category of processes to do with the weather: METEOROLOGICAL processes. They may be construed either existentially, e.g. *there was a storm / hurricane / wind / breeze / gale / shower / blizzard*, or as material events, e.g. *the wind's blowing, the sun's shining, the clouds are coming down.* Some are construed as relational attributives: *it's foggy / cloudy / misty / hot / humid / sunny / cold / frosty.* There is a last type which is unique, in that it has no participant in it. It is construed as *it* + a verb in present continuous: *it's raining / hailing / snowing / freezing / pouring / thundering.* The form *it* functions as Subject, like *there* in an existential process, but has no function in transitivity. On the other hand, the tense is clearly that of a material process. These clauses can be analysed as consisting of a single element, the Process; they are the limiting case of a material process clause.

It is precisely on the analogy of this analysis of meteorological processes as consisting only of the Process (or more accurately, as we shall see in a later section

5. They are the least distinct of all the six process types because they have no clearly defined characteristics of their own; rather they are partly like the material and partly like the mental.

of our discussion, as having the obligatory element MEDIUM conflated with the Process) that it is possible to represent the English form 'it's hurting' and its Greek translation equivalent *ponai* (an intransitive impersonal subjectless pain utterance) as also consisting of a Process in conflation with the Medium. Thus, as will be argued in the relevant section, in such constructions pain is configured as a meteorological process, with the word *it* (and the verb suffix in Greek) conflated with, i.e. indistinguishable from, the painful process itself.

Though from the standpoint of transitivity, each one of the six process types (material, behavioural, mental, verbal, relational and existential) has a grammar of its own, at another level of interpretation, namely, the 'ergative' pattern, they all have the same grammar, on the basis of just one variable. This variable relates to the source of the process: what it is that brought it about. The question at issue is: is the process brought about from within, or from outside? At this level of interpretation, the question is again how many participants there are, one or two. However, the variable here is not one of extension, as in the intransitive / transitive distinction, but rather one of causation. Some participant is engaged in a process; is the process brought about by that participant, or by some other entity? Compare *the boat sailed / Mary sailed the boat, the cloth tore / the nail tore the cloth, Tom's eyes closed / Tom closed his eyes.*

In the ergative pattern, every process has associated with it one obligatory participant, the MEDIUM, that is the key figure in that process. It is the entity through the medium of which the process is actualised, and without which there would be no process at all.[6] In the examples above, the Medium is *the boat, the cloth, his (Tom's) eyes.* Hence in a material process the Medium is equivalent to Actor in an intransitive clause and Goal in a transitive one.

According to the ergative option, the Process and the Medium together form the nucleus of an English clause. In addition, there may be another participant, the AGENT, i.e. an external cause represented as engendering the process from outside. A large number of processes may be structured either way: as involving Process + Medium only, i.e. as self-engendering, though in the real world there may have been some external agency involved, or as involving Medium plus Agent. Compare the clauses *the glass broke, the baby sat up*, to *the heat broke the glass, Jane sat the baby up.*

The Medium is the nodal participant throughout the system. Thus, it is not the doer nor the causer, but the one that is critically involved, in some way or other according to the particular nature of the process. The Agent is the external agency

6. Though the Medium is obligatory in all processes, for the sake of simplicity meteorological processes such as *it's raining* may be represented as having no Medium. However, as mentioned above, it would be more accurate to say that here the Medium is conflated with the Process.

where there is one. In a material process, it is the Actor – provided the process is one that has a Goal. In a mental process it is the Phenomenon.

The following figure illustrates how the functions can be matched in the various process types, if the ergative standpoint is used to complement the transitive one. For example, the ergative function Medium is equivalent:

in	material process	to	Actor (middle), Goal (effective)
	behavioural		Behaver
	mental		Senser
	verbal		Sayer (middle), Target (effective)
	attributive		Carrier
	identifying		Identified
	existential		Existent

The way the voice system works is as follows. A clause with no feature of 'agency' is neither active nor passive but MIDDLE. One with agency is non-MIDDLE, or EFFECTIVE, in voice. An effective clause is then either active or passive: active if Agent / Subject, passive if Medium / Subject. Strictly speaking, an effective clause has the feature 'agency' embodied rather than the structural function Agent, because this may be implicitly present, as in *the glass was broken*, where one can ask the question 'who by?'. By contrast, the middle clause *the glass broke* allows for one participant only, due to the absence of any (explicit or implicit) 'agency' feature.

I shall close this presentation by exemplifying the interrelation between transitivity functions and ergativity ones along the voice dimension, with respect to material processes. This will allow me to clarify a very subtle and important distinction between Actor and Agent that will be crucially used in the analysis of pain patterns. Thus, in a material process:

- if there is only one participant, in transitivity terms the clause will be intransitive and this single participant will be Actor, while in terms of voice the clause will be middle and the single participant will be Medium;
- if there are two participants, in transitivity terms the clause will be transitive with an Actor / Subject and a Goal, while in terms of voice the clause will be non-middle, i.e. effective. Here again there are two possibilities: active if Agent / Subject, passive if Medium / Subject.

The important distinction to capture here is that Agent is related to voice, while Actor is related to transitivity. Thus, Agent can only be present in effective (non-middle) clauses, i.e. clauses with two participants (in essence transitive clauses – whether active or passive), whereas Actor is necessarily present in material processes, whether intransitive or transitive. To conclude, Actor is also Agent in an effective, i.e. transitive clause, whereas Actor is Medium in a middle clause. Moreover, Goal is Medium in an effective clause.

Having provided a brief sketch of Halliday's understanding of the experiential function of the clause, we can proceed with the functional analysis of the lexicogrammar of pain in Greek and its juxtaposition with Halliday's paradigm of English pain expressions in the following chapters.

CHAPTER 5

Data analysis and general discussion

5.1 Introduction

In this chapter, following Gustafson's (1979: 151–152) suggested mode of analysis, we will be concerned with answering the '*what* kind' question addressed by Halliday (1998: 11), namely, "What type of element is 'pain'? Is it process, participant, or [...] a quality of something?" The identification of the predominant character of pain as process, participant, or quality, will provide us with an initial, yet vital, characterisation of its lexico-grammatical construal in Greek. In addition, our frequency counts will allow us to highlight this first impression of the mapping of pain onto Greek by revealing some of the key lexical items recurring in the doctor-patient discourse of pain. The insights we will gain from the analysis of our preliminary findings will enable us to engage in the thorough examination of the construal of pain as process and as participant in the subsequent chapters, thus providing answers to related '*which* kind' questions.

5.2 Pain: Process, participant or quality?

Halliday's understanding of the three components of a process, namely, the 'process' itself, the 'participants' and the 'circumstances' has been adopted in this study: I therefore assume the process to be typically realised by the verbal group of the clause, participants to be typically realised by nominal groups, and circumstances to be typically realised by adverbial groups or prepositional phrases. In addition, I assume 'qualities' to be realised by adjectival groups.

When we compute all the forms of the *ponao* 'I hurt' verb paradigm, all the nominal forms and the scarce adjectival ones that occurred in the doctor-patient dialogues, the frequency counts are quite revealing and provide, in relation to Greek, an indisputable answer to the crucial '*what* kind' question preoccupying Halliday as to how grammar construes pain as a domain of human experience.

Table 1 The lexico-grammatical construal of pain in Greek

Pain configurations		
Type	Frequency	
	Occurrences	%
Process (verb)	911	60.01
Participant (noun)	583	38.41
Quality (adjective)	24	1.58
Total	**1518**	**100.00**

Interestingly, while all verb occurrences are forms of the lexeme *ponao*, among the 583 instances of nominals, in addition to the 554 cases of the (morphologically simple) *ponos* forms, we observe three compounds, namely, *ponokefalos* 'headache' (13 cases), *mesopona* 'low back pain' / 'lumbago' (2 cases), and *skiloponos* 'dog pain', i.e. nasty pain (1 occurrence), two diminutives, i.e. *ponaki(a)* (8 cases) and *ponakos* (1 case), and additionally the nouns *isxialjia* 'sciatica' (2 cases) and *kolikos* 'colic' (2 cases) which are not morphologically related to *ponos*. Also, of the 24 adjectival constructions, 18 include the quasi-participle *ponemeno* 'sore' and 6 contain the adjective *epoδinos* 'painful' which is a more formal derivative of the archaic noun *oδini* 'pain' / 'dolour'.

The figures of Table 1 strongly reconfirm the claim initially put forward in the pilot study of Lascaratou and Hatzidaki (2002: 60) on the basis of a subset of the corpus data, namely, that "in the configuration of everyday experience Greek construes pain primarily as process (worded as a verb), secondarily as participant (worded as a noun), and only marginally as quality (worded as an adjective)." Despite the considerably larger size of the present corpus, i.e. 69,996 words vs. 47,464 words of the preliminary survey data, the relative frequencies of these three modes of pain construal are almost identical with the corresponding ones in the earlier sub-corpus (process: 60.01% vs. 62.63%, participant: 38.41% vs. 35.44%, and quality: 1.58% vs. 1.92%).

A central assumption in this study being that the understanding of pain as process, participant, quality or circumstance is related to the degree of involvement of the sufferer's self in the painful experience, it seems plausible to suggest that there is some gradience in the representation of this involvement, with the process expressing it *par excellence*, the participant following and quality and circumstance featuring at the other end.[1] Ultimately, it may be that the grammatical construal of pain reflects the nuclear character of verbs and nominals in propositions.

My understanding of the factors underlying the prevalence of verb constructions and the scarcity of adjectival ones in Greek pain utterances could be associated with Wierzbicka's (1992: 398–406) claim that Russian and English exhibit an interesting difference in the framing of emotions, namely, Russian favours a verbal pattern, while English opts for an adjectival one.[2] More specifically, comparing the way such emotional experiences as 'joy', 'sadness' or 'anger' are represented in these two languages, Wierzbicka suggests that in Russian they are often conceptualised as involving duration and implying quasi-voluntary inner activities and hence are often constructed as verbs, rather than adjectives. On the other hand, she argues, in English such experiences are more frequently linguistically realised as adjectives (e.g. *sad*, *afraid*, *angry*, *happy*, *glad*) and pseudo-participles (e.g. *pleased*, *worried*, *disgusted*, *ashamed*), which reflects their conceptualisation as passive states brought about by external and/or past causes.[3] Thus, for Wierzbicka the conceptualisation of emotions and their lexico-grammatical construal in a specific language are interdependent.

In addition, Wierzbicka's claim that, when emotions are realised as verbs, they tend to be expressed as part of an action with externally observable manifestations, suggests that for her the verbal pattern in the construction of emotions actually constitutes the most dynamic linguistic expression of emotions. In other words,

1. My understanding of 'involvement' is essentially captured in the working definition provided by Inchaurralde (1997: 135): "By emotional involvement in this paper I understand affective proximity or detachment."

2. Though I believe that a culturally based approach to the language of pain in Greek would contribute to the understanding of the subtleties of this domain of human experience, it is beyond the scope of the present study to engage in a systematic consideration of cultural factors related to pain. Without embarking on such a venture, I shall, nevertheless, selectively refer to those aspects of culturally oriented research into the language of pain and emotions in general, in which my intuitions find support with regard to the lexico-grammatical construal of pain.

3. Pavlenko's (2002: 207) quantitative and qualitative analyses of American and Russian narrative corpora fully support Wierzbicka's views, suggesting "that 'the reading of the body' is not a culture- and language-free experience, but is shaped by cultural, social, and linguistic forces, as well as by individual differences." Pavlenko's study (*ibid.*: 224–225) demonstrates that while both speech communities may frame emotions as states, this discursive construction is clearly secondary in the Russian corpus, where emotions are predominantly constructed as an active process. Thus, while American monolingual participants emphasise the passive – and even induced – state aspect of emotions, monolingual Russian participants consistently exhibit a preference for framing emotions as an active process through the use of imperfective verbs, whose meaning is "more immediate and refers to experiencing, processing, and dealing with particular emotions, most often 'suffering them through.'"

according to Wierzbicka, when Russian people express emotions, their patterns of behaviour are linguistically more 'active', 'dynamic', 'loaded', 'theatrical', and 'public', compared to those of English people, this 'linguistic acting out' being both reflected in and determined by the inherently more actional features of verbs.

I believe that my understanding of verbal pain avowals in Greek as belonging to the most expressive forms of pain language – with certain patterns often functioning as interjections (which sit between verbal avowals and actual cries / groans / screams) – and Wierzbicka's analysis of verbal utterances of emotions in Russian essentially converge in that they both see verb forms as bringing out the experiencer's active involvement in the emotion or pain process (see section 6.4 for relevant discussion). The prevalence of verb constructions observed in the Greek doctor-patient corpus of the present study suggests that, in expressing a painful condition, Greek speakers typically prefer the more direct, dramatic, and dynamic framing of pain provided by verbs. It would be extremely interesting, of course, to examine if Greek also steadily favours the verbal pattern in the construction of emotions in general. Though I expect that my findings on pain could be associated with Greek cultural attitudes along the same lines that Wierzbicka interprets Russian and English emotion data, I cannot help considering the potential role played by an additional factor, namely, that both Greek and Russian are morphologically rich languages with complex verb paradigms enabling their speakers to express delicate nuances of processes. These issues will be taken up in the subsequent discussion of my findings in terms of the grammatical features of the various modes of pain construal within Halliday's functional paradigm, whereby I will be able to further refine my analysis.

Finally, the extremely limited number of occurrences (i.e. 24) of the only two adjectival forms denoting 'sore / painful', namely, *ponemenos* and *epoδinos*, observed in all the material motivated the decision not to include any account of the understanding of pain as quality and to focus on its construal as process and participant.

It seems useful, however, to mention here a few observations regarding the collected adjectival patterns. Thus, in all its occurrences in the corpus, 18 in total, the quasi-participle *ponemeno* 'sore' is used as an adjectival attributive modifier of a noun denoting a body part, typically one that has recently undergone surgery, rather than as an adjectival predicate in a copula construction. It was observed that in most of the cases the body part is not explicitly mentioned but, instead, it is referred to by means of its modifier *ponemeno*. Consider the following:[4]

(1) D: vale *to ponemeno to poδi* bros, pame, *to ponemeno* ipa bros. eki.

4. In the extracts from the doctor-patient dialogues, D introduces the doctor / medical expert, P stands for the patient, and in the very few cases where there is a third person, usually a relative, who takes part in the dialogue, I have used R (relative) to denote him/her.

put-IMP:2SG the sore-ACC the leg-ACC in front let's go-IMP:1PL the sore-ACC say-PST:1SG in front there
'Put *the sore leg* in front, let's go, *the sore one*, I said, in front. There.'

(2) P: aaax! ma mu lete olo to aristero *to ponemeno*.
ouch but I-GEN say-PRS:2PL all-the time the left-ACC the sore-ACC
'Ouch! But you keep telling me "the left one, *the sore one*" all the time.'

(3) D: ela, pame, isa isa, ke pame. brosta to xirurjimeno, e? *to ponemeno*. pame eki. bravo!
come-IMP:2SG let's go-IMP:1PL straight straight and let's go-IMP:1PL in front the operated-ACC yeah the sore-ACC let's go-IMP:1PL well-done
'Come on, let's go, straight ahead, and let's go. The operated one in front, yeah? *The sore one.* Let's go, there you are. Well done!'

On the other hand, the adjective *epoδinos* 'painful', which occurred in a single dialogue, appears 4 times as an adjectival modifier of a noun denoting a sensation / feeling and twice as an adjectival predicate of a syntactic object:

(4) D: orea. ara afti i esθisi, as to pume, ine ena fisiolojiko i ine *epoδino sinesθima*?
good therefore this the sensation-NOM let's say-IMP:1PL be-PRS:3SG a normal-NOM or be-PRS:3SG painful-NOM feeling-NOM
'Good. Therefore, is this sensation, let's say, a normal or a *painful feeling*?'

P: *epoδino*.
painful-NOM
'(It's a) *painful* (one).'

D: ine *epoδino*. δilaδi, ja na boresume na to orioθetisume liγaki ke na to valume se mja vasi, exete *epoδini tin esθisi* tis plirosis?
be-PRS:3SG painful-NOM that-is in order to-PARTCL can-PRS:1PL to-ARTCL it-ACC delimitate-PRS:1PL a-little and to-PARTCL it-ACC put-PRS:1PL on a basis-ACC, have-PRS:2PL painful-ACC the sensation-ACC of filling-up-GEN
'It's *painful*. To be more explicit so that we can somehow delimitate it and put it on a (proper) basis, do you experience *the sensation* of filling up (of the cyst) as being *painful*?'

P: akrivos.
precisely
'Precisely.'

D: ke…
and
'And…'

P: ...ke *epoδino* ke *tin apovoli.*
and painful-ACC and the discharge-ACC
'...and also *the discharge* as being *painful.*'

5.3 Key lexical items and their frequencies

Before we move on to the analysis of the various constructions where pain is construed as a process or a participant, it is worth considering the relative frequency of some lexical items that occurred in the data, as I believe that they are representative of the particular type of discourse from which the data were derived. What is more, the high frequency of certain lexemes as well as specific collocations will indicate to us some significant aspects of the discourse context within which pain is expressed and/or described.

Looking first at the corpus as a whole (69,996 words), i.e. both doctors' and patients' data, we observe that, among verb forms, the third-person singular *ponai* 'it hurts' / 'it's hurting' is the most frequent lexical (i.e. not functional) word and the most frequent verb (384 occurrences) after the delexical *ine* 'is' / 'are' (964 cases). It should be noted that the frequency figure of *ponai* covers a variety of constructions where this form occurs, i.e. transitive, intransitive, personal, and impersonal, with reference to a body part or with no such reference. The next most frequent verb forms are the first-person plural *pame* 'let's go' / 'we go' (274 instances) and the first-person singular *exo* 'I have' (267 cases) followed by the third-person singular *exi* '(s)he / it has' (234 occurrences).

The high frequency of *pame* can be explained by the fact that in most cases it is an imperative, meaning 'let's go / try together', used as a form of encouragement by medical experts in their attempt to persuade patients to carry out activities that they may hesitate to attempt for fear that they may undergo pain, e.g. walk after surgery or make particular movements with an arm in pain. The following is a characteristic example:

(5) ja *pame* mazi... *pame.* etsi bravo, *pame.* oso pai. ela, ke kato... *pame*... orea... δinata.
let's go-IMP:1PL together go-IMP:1PL like-this well-done go-IMP:1PL as-much-as go-PRS:3SG come-IMP:2SG and down go-IMP:1PL fine strongly
'*Let's go* together... *let's go.* That's it, well done, *let's go.* As far as it'll go. Come on, (move it) downwards too... *let's go*... fine... with all your strength.'

It is not surprising that the forms *exo* and *exi* have high frequencies, given that the verb *exo* is used as an auxiliary in the formation of (present and past) perfect tenses. In addition, *exo* + nominal structures are quite common in Greek. In particular, as we shall see in more detail in the relevant section 8.2.1, *exo* + *ponos* constructions are used alongside structures containing the verbs *esθanome* 'I feel' and *njoθo* 'I feel' with *ponos* as their object. Moreover, *exo* + *ponos* constructions may be construed as either relational, if *exo* is analysed as a semantically empty, linking verb (see Theophanopoulou-Kontou, 1988 and Moser, 1993), or as possessive, if *exo* is understood as primarily possessive (see Veloudis, 2003 and Nikiforidou, 1991). In addition to *ponos,* in the patients' data the form *exo* also collocates with other nouns showing discomfort or distress, e.g. *enoxlisi* 'annoyance', *provlima* 'problem', *kataθlipsi* 'depression', *plakosi* 'anguish', *aδjaθesia* 'malaise', *aiδia* 'nausea', as well as with nouns denoting various health problems or illnesses, such as *astaθia* 'instability', *eksanθima* 'rash', *spasmi* 'spasms', *piesi* 'blood pressure', *elkos* 'ulcer', *zaxaro* 'diabetes', *(δisko)kili* 'displaced disc' and *skoliosi* 'scoliosis'. Thus, *exo* + nominal constructions prove to be quite productive in the expression of bodily sensations and psychological conditions:[5]

(6) pote pote, *exo ekini tin tin kataθlipsi, ekino ton iδrota, ekino to…*
occasionally have-PRS:1SG that the the depression-ACC that the sweating-ACC that the
'Occasionally, *I have that that depression, that sweating, that…*'

(7) akoma ke tora pu sizitame, *eyo exo tin enoxlisi mu* eδo pera.
even and now that talk-PRS:1PL I-NOM have-PRS:1SG the discomfort-ACC my here
'Even now that we are talking, *I have my feeling of discomfort* here.'

(8) lipon, *exo xronia provlima me ta kokala, me tin plati,* me ponai.
well I have-PRS:1SG years-ACC problems-ACC with the bones-ACC, with the back-ACC, I-ACC hurt-PRS:3SG
'Well, *for years I've had problems with my bones, with my back,* it hurts me.'

Notably, the first-person singular form *boro* 'I can' is also quite frequent, numbering 185 cases, of which 157, i.e. 84.86%, occurred in the patients' material. The most interesting aspect of clauses containing the form *boro* is that overall, in both doctors' and patients' data, they are predominantly negative ones, their frequency among patients' *boro* utterances amounting to 120 cases, i.e. 76.43%. Therefore, rather than expressing possibility or ability, the majority of patients' *boro* clauses actually denote impossibility and inability. I suggest that this strong tendency of

5. Theophanopoulou-Kontou (personal communication) points out the existence of additional *exo* constructions, such as *exo* + *xara* 'joy' / *lipi* 'sorrow', *kefia* / 'high spirits', *ginia* 'bad luck' / *tis mavres mu* 'the (my) blues', all of which express a (psychological) state, like the corresponding *ime* 'I am' patterns, e.g. *ime sta kefia mu* 'I am in high spirits, *ime stis mavres mu* 'I am in low spirits / I've got the blues'.

the form *boro* to collocate with the negative particle *δen* in patients' speech should be interpreted as a significant indication of the feelings of disability, powerlessness, weakness, helplessness, vulnerability, and defenselessness experienced by the sufferer. If we examine the various verbs of the *na* clauses complementing the sequence *δen* + *boro*, we shall gain some insight into the main activities that patients feel incapable of carrying out as a consequence of their painful condition. Thus, we observe that *δen* + *boro* is followed by such complement clauses as:

(9) *na anapnefso* '(to) breathe'
(10) *na paro anasa* '(to) take a breath'
(11) *n' andekso* '(to) endure'
(12) *na katalavo* '(to) understand'
(13) *na volefto* '(to) feel at ease'
(14) *na oriso ton pono* '(to) have control over pain'
(15) *na kano tipota* '(to) do anything'
(16) *na katso* '(to) remain seated'
(17) *na kiniθo* '(to) move'
(18) *na mino isia* '(to) keep my body straight'
(19) *na miliso* '(to) speak'
(20) *na oδijiso* '(to) drive'
(21) *na perpatiso* '(to) walk'
(22) *na staθo kaθolu* '(to) stand up at all'
(23) *na stereoθo sta poδia mu* '(to) be steady on my feet'
(24) *na pjaso tipota* '(to) hold anything'
(25) *na jiriso to kefali eki* '(to) turn my head there'
(26) *na t' angikso kaθolu* '(to) touch it at all'
(27) *na to sikoso* '(to) lift it'
(28) *na to kuniso* '(to) move it'

Hence, these negative feelings are mostly associated with the patient's power to survive, as well as to endure, understand, and control his pain, his ability to move his body or some body part in space or engage in some everyday activity.

This interpretation gains support from the observation that in as many as 43 of the 120 *δen* + *boro* structures (35.83%, i.e. over one third), there is no *na*- 'to-' clausal complement. In fact, the absence of a complement to which the lack of ability would be 'extended' makes the feelings of powerlessness and weakness seem even more intense, in the sense that these feelings are not associated with any particular activity but, rather, they are stated as a general condition, something like an exclamation of despair. Let us look at some representative examples:

(29) otan ime akiniti ponao poli, *δen boro*.
when be-PRS:1SG still-NOM hurt-PRS:1SG a-lot not can-PRS:1SG
'When I don't move I hurt a lot, *I can't*.'

(30) *δen boro*, ponane ta poδia mu.
not can-PRS:1SG hurt-PRS:3PL the legs-NOM my
'*I can't*, my legs are hurting.'

(31) aaax, *δen boro*, θa me ksekanis.
ah not can-PRS:1SG will I-ACC tear-apart-PRS:2SG
'Ah, *I can't*, you will tear me apart.'

(32) ax, ax, *δen boro*, jatre.
ah ah not can-PRS:1SG doctor-VOC
'Ah, ah, *I can't*, doctor.'

This negative collocation should be associated with the fact that the negative word *δen* is the fifth most frequent form – after the exclamation *a* 'ah', the article *to* 'the', the conjunction *ke* 'and', and the particle *na* 'to' – in the patients' subcorpus. This issue will be taken up in our presentation of some collocations of the negative particles *δen* and *mi*(*n*) below.

Resuming our presentation of the most frequent verbs, it should be observed that the next most frequent forms are the imperative of *erxome* 'I come', i.e. *ela* (176 cases), and the subjunctive of the verb *le*(*γ*)*o* 'say', namely, *po* (164 cases). With regard to *ela*, it is suggested that its numerous occurrences can be understood in, more or less, the same way as the high frequency of *pame*, that is, as a form of encouragement on the part of the medical staff. I cannot help observing that both *ela* and *pame* are imperatives of motion verbs, 'come' and 'go', respectively, as if the encouragement addressed to patients is linguistically realised by means of verbs whereby health care experts urge pain sufferers to move and, thus, overcome the immobilisation that pain imposes on them. Consider example (5) above where *pame* and *ela* typically co-occur. As for the high frequency of *po*, it is not surprising in a discourse type such as that of our doctor-patient interviews, considering that patients are asked to put into words various aspects of their painful experiences.

After *ela* comes the first-person singular *ponao* 'I hurt' / 'I'm hurting' with 153 instances, by means of which pain avowals are typically configured. The central role of this particular pain expression will concern us in our discussion of the construal of pain as process (sections 6.3 and 6.4).

Another interesting observation is that the first-person singular *ksero* 'I know' numbers 127 occurrences, the majority of which (98, i.e. 77.16%) appeared in patients' utterances, mostly collocating with the negative particle *δen* (65/98, i.e.

66.33%). I suggest that in the context of our doctor-patient dialogues, the sequence *δen + ksero* can be interpreted as an alternative, almost synonymous, expression to *δen + boro*, in the sense that it is understood as bringing out the sufferer's feeling of ignorance as to how he could handle his painful experience which again amounts to feelings of powerlessness, helplessness, etc. In other words, for the sufferer 'to know' means 'to be able to' and, conversely, 'not to know' means 'to be unable to' come to grips with his situation. This understanding is further highlighted by the occurrence of about 20 utterances where the pattern *δen + ksero* is not followed by any nominal or clausal complement but, rather, it functions like an afterthought, an introspective comment, a murmur of despair (see the discussion of similar *δen + boro* utterances above). There are also cases where the sequence *δen + ksero* reflects the sufferer's inability or ignorance as to how he could put the painful experience into words in his attempt to deal with it and communicate it (express or describe it) to others. Consider:

(33) me ponai. *δen ksero.*
I-ACC hurt-PRS:3SG not know-PRS:1SG
'It's hurting me. *I don't know.*'

(34) *δen ksero* kale… *δen ksero.*
not know-PRS:1SG dear-VOC not know-PRS:1SG
'*I don't know* my dear… *I don't know.*'

(35) *δen ksero*, etsi me pniji ena prama.
not know-PRS:1SG like-this I-ACC strangle-PRS:3SG a thing-NOM
'*I don't know*, it is as if something is strangling me.'

Other verb forms which occurred quite frequently are: the first-person singular *θelo* 'I want' in 93 utterances, the first-person singular *esθanome* 'I feel' with 62 cases and 36 other forms of the same lexeme (i.e. 98 instances in all), the second-person singular / plural *njoθis* / *njoθete* 'you feel' with 94 occurrences, plus 13 cases of the first-person *njoθo* and 10 more cases of other forms of the same verbal lexeme (i.e. 117 in all). Constructions containing the verbs *esθanome* and *njoθo* will be considered in the analysis of *ponos* 'pain' configurations (section 8.2.1).

Let us now examine some of the nouns that were observed in the material. By far the most frequent noun form is the nominative singular *ponos* 'pain' numbering 280 instances, while the accusative singular *pono* occurred in 191 cases. In fact, in the patients' data the accusative *pono* is the next most frequent noun form after the nominative *ponos*. It is quite revealing that, whether we look at all the material together or at the patients' data only, the picture of the relative frequency of the nominative *ponos* and the accusative *pono* that we get is close to identical in both cases, namely, about 60% for *ponos* and 40% for *pono*. What these figures tell us is that in our authentic Greek dialogues, the noun for pain is configured as the syntactic subject in the majority of utterances, whereas it is construed as the syntactic object in the minority of the constructions where it occurs. In terms of the participant roles that pain as thing can be assigned, the frequency counts indicate that in the majority of clauses *ponos* will be configured as Actor (in material middle processes), both Actor and Agent (in material effective processes), and Carrier (in relational-attributive processes). On the other hand, in the minority of clauses, *pono* will be understood as Phenomenon (in mental processes) or Attribute (in relational-possessive processes). Though in a later section (7.3) we will be discussing in detail the types of figure where *ponos* as an entity enters and the associated participant roles whereby it is configured, I cannot help observing at this early stage of the analysis that pain seems to be construed as a rather dynamic participant. This understanding of pain will become more evident when we come to metaphorical *ponos* nominal constructions, where the actional / agentive interpretation of *ponos* will prove to be crucial (sections 8.2.2 and 8.2.3).

Though, as we shall see in our analysis of the construal of pain as process, the sufferer's body part is configured as a participant in only about one fifth of such clauses (section 6.3), it is worth looking at the various parts of the body that were most frequently referred to in the material. I am, of course, aware that my findings are biased, given that a great amount of my material comprises dialogues with patients suffering from musculoskeletal problems. Thus, the most frequent word denoting a body part is *poδi(a)* 'leg(s)' / 'foot(feet)' with 311 instances. It is also, in fact, the next most frequent noun after *ponos* in all the material. In addition to *poδi(a)*, the following names for body parts were also found in considerable numbers, the figures indicating their occurrences in descending order of frequency: *xeri(a)* 'arm(s)' / 'hand(s)' (132), *plati* 'back' (77), *mesi* 'low back' (74), *kefali* 'head' (55), *yonato* 'knee' (51), *yofos/i* 'hip(s)' (22), and *δaxtilo/a* 'finger(s)'(22).[6]

Unlike body parts, which are not systematically mentioned in pain utterances, locative adverbial phrases are quite abundant in the material. In particular, 504 out of the 875 instances of the adverbial *eδo* 'here', which is the tenth most frequent word in the entire corpus, and 176 out of the 413 instances of the adverbial *eki* 'there' are used, either by medical experts or patients, to identify the location of pain. Besides, the noun *simio/a* 'point(s)', which is also employed to indicate where pain is located, appears in 68 cases. Our data analysis will show that the tendency to identify pain in terms of its location correlates more with its construal as an

6. Other body parts occurred quite marginally, such as *karδia* 'heart' (13), *stomaxi* 'stomach' (13), *nefro/a* 'kidney(s)' (9), *omos/i* 'shoulder(s)' (9), *omoplati* 'shoulder blade' (8), *endero/a* 'intestine(s)' (3), and *sikoti* 'liver' (3).

entity rather than as a process. In fact, as we shall see, location is one of the basic syntactico-semantic features of pain as thing (see section 7.2).

Having observed that negative utterances are quite common in the material overall, i.e. in both doctors' and patients' data computed together, I think it useful to close this presentation of the most frequent lexical items in the corpus, by mentioning some negative collocations in the patients' subcorpus.

Our first observation is that in patients' speech the negative particle *δe(n)* is the fifth most frequent word with 819 occurrences, while the particle *mi(n)* is found in 103 cases, which means that there is a total of 922 negative clauses. Of the 819 *δe(n)* utterances, in 163, which represent almost one fifth (i.e. 19.90%) of them, *δe(n)* collocates with various forms of the verb *boro*, which has already been interpreted as an indication of the patients' feelings of powerlessness. What is more, of these 163 negative clauses as many as 120, i.e. 73.62%, contain the first-person singular form, while, as we saw above, 43 (26.38%) are *δen* + *boro* constructions taking no complement at all. Moreover, in the 65 clauses where *δen* collocates with the first-person singular verb form *ksero*, we observe similar cases of elliptical *δen* + *ksero* sequences.

Though their frequencies are not considerable, there are some cases of collocations of *δen* with such verbs as *exo* 'I have', *andexo* 'I endure', 'I tolerate', and *kimame* 'I sleep', which are typical representations of the sufferer's condition. For example:

(36) *δen exo to kurajo.*
not have-PRS:1SG the courage-ACC
'*I don't have the courage.*'

(37) ala *δen exo psixi.*
but not have-PRS:1SG soul-ACC
'But *I have lost heart.*'

(38) *δen andexo*, aaa.
not endure-PRS:1SG ah
'*I can't take it*, ah, ah, ah.'

(39) *δen kimame kaθolu.*
not sleep-PRS:1SG at-all
'*I don't sleep at all.*'

Finally, there are also 8 cases where *δen* is used in elliptical structures on its own, i.e. without being followed by a verb, hence, functioning like a vague negative comment.

Most instances of the other negative particle, namely, *mi(n)*, are collocations with imperative forms, whereby the patient urges the medical expert not to do to him something that is unpleasant or painful.

(40) *min to xtipas*, jati ponai, ponai… pa pa pa…
not it-ACC hit-PRS:2SG because hurt-PRS:3SG hurt-PRS:3SG ouch ouch ouch
'*Don't hit it*, because it hurts, it hurts… ouch ouch ouch…'

(41) *min mu kanis alo*, δen andexo.
not I-GEN do-PRS:2SG any-more not endure-PRS:1SG
'*Don't do that to me anymore*, I can't take it.'

(42) *mi* re x, *mi me θanatonis* toso.
not man not I-ACC kill-PRS:2SG so-much
'*Don't*, you man, *don't you kill me* that much.'

Moreover, *mi* without the euphonic final *n*, is also used as a negative exclamation aiming at stopping the interlocutor from doing something. As such, it often co-occurs with exclamations of pain as well as with the third-person impersonal *ponai* form, which, as will be claimed, often functions as an interjection. Consider the following:

(43) oxi jatre, jatre, *mi* sas parakalo.
no doctor-VOC doctor-VOC not you-ACC:PL beg-PRS:1SG
'No doctor, doctor, please *don't*.'

(44) ponai. *mi*! a! eki!
hurt-PRS:3SG:IMPERS not ah there
'It's hurting. *Don't*! Ah! There!'

(45) *mi*, *mi*, *mi*. ponai.
not not not hurt-PRS:3SG:IMPERS
'*Don't*, *don't*, *don't*. It's hurting.'

In this chapter, on the basis of frequency counts, it has been possible to provide solid empirical evidence in support of the characterisation of the lexico-grammatical construal of pain in Greek as primarily verbal (denoting a process), secondarily nominal (denoting a participant), and only marginally adjectival (denoting a quality). As the thorough analysis of the collected pain patterns in Chapter 6 will show, my interpretation of the predominantly verbal construal of pain in Greek essentially coincides with Wierzbicka's claim that the framing of emotions as verbs reflects their understanding as active, inner, quasi-voluntary, processual events. Moreover, the frequency counts applied onto our data have revealed the central role played by certain lexical items recurring in the doctor-patient dialogues, such as the noun *ponos* 'pain', the verb form *ponai* 'it hurts' / 'it's hurting', the verb *exo* 'have', the negative particles *δen* and *mi*(*n*) frequently co-occurring with the verb forms *boro* 'I can' and *ksero* 'I know', and finally the locative adverbials *eδo* 'here' and *eki* 'there', used in identification of pain location.

CHAPTER 6

The construal of pain as process

6.1 Introduction

In this chapter, I shall examine the Greek structural configurations of pain as process in my attempt to answer the '*which* kind' question concerning the processual construal of pain in everyday experience.

Alongside the examination of the lexico-grammatical properties of the relevant structures, I shall also be concerned with their expressive vs. descriptive function in communicating pain. The data analysis will show that, among the patterns where pain is configured as a process through various forms of the *ponao* 'I hurt' verb paradigm, some particular constructions have a stronger expressive rather than descriptive function. In the light of the IASP definition of pain adopted in this study (see section 2.2.1.1), namely as *both a sensory and emotional* experience, I shall be able to propose a schematic representation for my intuitions by mapping onto pain behaviour Foolen's (1997) analysis of the twofold communication channel of emotions, i.e. paralinguistic manifestations vs. verbal utterances. What is more, I shall suggest an answer to a critical question explicitly posed by Foolen himself as inevitably emerging from his own exposition.

6.2 Foolen's account of the communication of emotions and pain behaviour

The main assumption put forth in Foolen's (1997) proposal is that though ideas (cognition) are verbally expressed through words and paralinguistically through signs, emotions (affect) are typically voiced through cries and communicated paralinguistically through gestures. This assumption, Foolen warns us, should not be misinterpreted as implying that emotions cannot be communicated through the verbal channel.

It is a further distinction that he makes to support his view that may be invoked to shed light on pain communication: he argues that emotion can be externalised in two qualitatively different ways, namely, the direct way, i.e. through the non-verbal and paralinguistic channel, and the indirect way, through verbalisations. Foolen justifies his characterisation of the verbal channel of emotion as *in-*

direct by assuming that "in a verbal utterance the *conceptualization* of the feeling is communicated" (*ibid.*: 20), rather than the emotion itself. He proposes the following diagram to represent his understanding of (a) the difference between the way ideas (cognition) and emotions (affect) are communicated, and (b) the two channels (direct and indirect) whereby emotions are externalised (*ibid.*: 20):

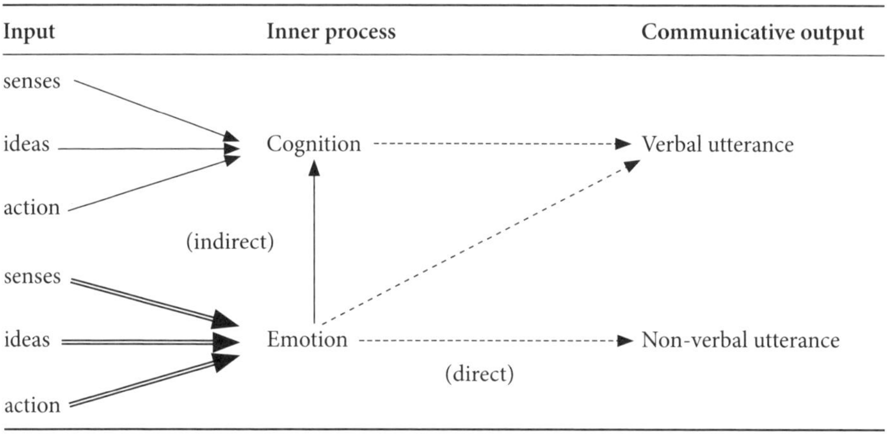

Figure 1 Foolen's (1997) suggested illustration of the communication of cognitive and emotional content

Having made these fine distinctions, Foolen finally addresses a very plausible question: does the linguistic expression of emotion *always* constitute an indirect channel of communication, or can we assume that there are also verbal utterances directly related to emotion, i.e. without the intermediary step of conceptualisation? This third way of externalising emotion is schematically indicated by the dotted line that directly links emotion to verbal utterance in his figure.

Mapping the proposed analysis of the function of pain utterances in terms of a 'primitive reaction – linguistic manifestation (expression and/or description)' continuum (Lascaratou and Hatzidaki, 2002: 55–56, 71) onto Foolen's (1997) account of the communication of emotion, I shall assume that automatic pain reactions, such as cries / groans / screams, correspond to Foolen's direct, non-verbal mode of communicating emotion and, hence, I shall identify them with one of the two extreme poles of the continuum. I shall reserve the other end of the spectrum for the cognitively motivated indirect channel, associated with objectifying descriptive nominal *ponos* 'pain' constructions, in particular those metaphorically structured (see Lascaratou and Marmaridou, 2005), assuming with Foolen that their conceptualisation precedes their verbalisation, i.e. that they constitute an indirect (*via* cognition) channel of externalising pain (see Chapter 8).

As an answer to the question Foolen poses, I shall venture to propose that the direct linguistic expression of pain in Greek can sometimes be identified with specific forms of its construal as process, namely, intransitive (either first-person *ponao* 'I hurt' / 'I'm hurting' or impersonal third-person *ponai* 'it hurts' / 'it's hurting') pain avowals, when these have an exclamatory function, i.e. when they function like interjections, with which they are actually observed to co-occur or alternate quite frequently in the corpus. Interjections being the linguistic signs positioned most closely to the proposed expressive pole of pain behaviour (which comprises cries / groans / screams, i.e. automatic non-linguistic pain reactions), I suggest that the linguistic forms functioning like interjections could assume a position next to them. This interpretation of the particular pain avowals in the light of Foolen's understanding of a potential direct verbal mode of emotion communication allows me not only to put forth the expressive function that I assume them to have but also to represent it schematically.

6.3 General characteristics of pain as process

Let us now examine in detail the various constructions whereby pain is construed as process that were collected in the Greek doctor-patient dialogues. As a working paradigm I will be using the one proposed by Halliday (1998: 16–17) according to the general theory of transitivity and the description of the English transitivity system presented in Halliday (1985/94, Ch. 5) and Matthiessen (1995b, Ch. 4). For ease of presentation, both the Greek structures observed in the data and Halliday's English paradigm of pain as 'process' are to be found in Appendix A. After presenting some general characteristic properties of these structural configurations of pain, I shall elaborate on the details of the type of process and structural functions associated with every expression.

It is necessary to mention here two morpho-syntactic issues that were taken into consideration in the computation of the frequency counts applied to the data. The first one is related to the possibility of suppressing the subject pronoun of Greek verbs due to their rich morphological marking, whereby the verb suffix indicates the person and the number of the subject, i.e. it functions as a 'copy' of the grammatical subject.[1] Thus, rather than compute subjectless structures separately, it was judged appropriate to include them under their corresponding subjectful ones.

1. In Generative Grammar terms, Greek is a pro-drop language (see Philippaki-Warburton, 1987, 1992).

Table 1 Pain as process: Verb configurations observed in the corpus

Verb configurations				
Pain expression	**Type of structure**	**Pat %**	**Doc %**	**Total %**
ponao / ponas (eδo)? 'I hurt / I'm hurting (here)' 'do you hurt / are you hurting (here)?'	intransitive-personal	41.23	53.94	**46.82**
ponai (eδo) 'it hurts / it's hurting (here)'	intransitive-impersonal	20.12	19.08	**19.66**
to xeri mu (mu) ponai 'my arm hurts / my arm's hurting (in me)'	intransitive + body part	15.14	14.25	**14.75**
me ponai (eδo) 'it hurts me / it's hurting me (here)'	transitive-impersonal	8.57	4.07	**6.59**
to xeri mu me ponai 'my arm's hurting me'	transitive + body part	8.96	2.29	**6.03**
afto ponai 'that hurts'	intransitive-agentive (*afto* other than body part)	3.59	2.04	**2.90**
afto me ponai 'that's hurting me'	transitive (*afto* other than body part)	1.59	3.31	**2.35**
me ponas / se ponao? 'you're hurting me'/ 'am I hurting you?'	transitive-personal	0.80	1.02	**0.90**
Total		100.0	100.0	**100.0**

The second issue concerns the absence of a simple present – present continuous morphological distinction in Greek, parallel to the one that exists in English, which would facilitate the mapping of the Greek data onto the corresponding English expressions. The fact that such a morphologically marked distinction is not relevant for Greek does not mean that the forms are ambiguous for the Greek native speaker, but rather that one must rely heavily on the context to interpret them. Hence, the form *ponao* may be interpreted as either 'I hurt' or 'I'm hurting', the expression *to xeri mu ponai* as either 'my arm hurts' or 'my arm's hurting', the intransitive-impersonal *ponai* as either 'it hurts' or 'it's hurting', while the transitive-impersonal *me ponai* as either 'it hurts me' or 'it's hurting me'. In all the frequency counts of the present study it was decided not to attempt any finer computations of these present tense forms on the grounds of context-based interpretations, with a single exception: only in Table 3 (see below) was an attempt made at refining the counts, with a view to gaining some insights into the real-life distinction between chronic and acute pain.

Table 2 Pain as process: Five most frequent verb configurations observed in the corpus

	Verb configurations			
Pain expression	**Type of structure**	**Pat %**	**Doc %**	**Total %**
ponao / ponas (eδo)? 'I hurt / I'm hurting (here)' 'do you hurt / are you hurting (here)?'	intransitive-personal	43.86	57.61	**49.88**
ponai (eδo) 'it hurts / it's hurting (here)'	intransitive-impersonal	21.40	20.38	**20.95**
to xeri mu (mu) ponai 'my arm hurts / my arm's hurting (in me)'	intransitive + body part	16.10	15.22	**15.71**
me ponai (eδo) 'it hurts me / it's hurting me (here)'	transitive-impersonal	9.11	4.35	**7.03**
to xeri mu me ponai 'my arm's hurting me'	transitive + body part	9.53	2.44	**6.43**
Total		100.0	100.0	**100.0**

These amendments provide us with the eight constructions figuring in Table 1 in descending order of frequency, as they were observed in both patients' and doctors' data. We observe that of the total of these eight configurations of pain as process that were collected in the material, three occurred quite marginally, namely, *afto ponai* 'that hurts',[2] (*afto*) *me ponai* 'that's hurting me',[3] and *me ponas* / *se ponao*? 'you're hurting me' / 'am I hurting you?', amounting together to only 6.15%. Though

2. As we shall see in the subsequent analysis of this structure (section 6.4), *afto* does not refer to a body part but instead it may be an external inanimate entity, such as an object, e.g. a medical instrument, or a process, e.g. a pain-inducing activity.

3. See note 2 above.

these three structures will be included in some more frequency counts to be discussed below, I suggest that it would be useful to ignore them at this point and look at the relative frequencies of the other five more frequent construals of pain computed on their own in Table 2.

It is striking that in both doctors' and patients' data the five statistically most prevalent constructions follow the same descending order of frequency, with the intransitive-personal *ponao* / *ponas* (*eδo*)? 'I hurt / I'm hurting (here)' / 'do you hurt / are you hurting (here)?' by far the most frequent one, representing, in fact, half of them (49.88%),[4] and *to xeri mu me ponai* 'my arm's hurting me' occurring incredibly infrequently (6.43%).

Although the frequencies of these structures are more or less evenly distributed between patients' and doctors' data, some interesting differences emerge if the patients' and the doctors' figures are compared. Thus, for example, the first-person *ponao* covers the 43.86% of patients' utterances, while the corresponding second-person (singular / plural) *ponas* / *ponate* in doctors' speech is considerably more frequent, i.e. 57.61%.

The majority of *ponas* / *ponate* instances (124 out of 212, i.e. 58.49%) are used in doctors' interrogative utterances – either yes/no questions, e.g. *ponas eδo*? 'are you hurting here?', or wh-questions, such as *pu ponas*? 'where do you hurt / are you hurting?', *pote ponas*? 'when do you hurt / are you hurting?'. Hence, it seems that this very high frequency of the intransitive-personal *ponas* / *ponate* can be accounted for by the fact that this form lends itself to being used by medical experts when first encountering the patient, i.e. in order to collect information about the cause, origin, and location of his pain. I suggest that, before actually being able to identify a patient's pain in terms of a number of properties, the doctor is confronted with the patient's suffering self as a whole entity seeking for relief, rather than with the treatment of a suffering body part as a distinct entity. Moreover, as regards the patient's very frequent use of *ponao*, it seems that, in addition to func-

4. I wish to note here that it was pointed out to me by a colleague that the English intransitive personal form *I hurt* / *I'm hurting* is not registered by the *Oxford English Dictionary* in the sense of 'I experience / I'm experiencing pain', nor does it occur in everyday language, even though it is one of Halliday's (1998) examples. Indeed, this seems to be the case, the two examples to be found in the *Compact Oxford English Dictionary* (1991), namely, *I'm sorry you're hurting* (1970) and *When I heard that… I thought I'd be hurting* (1972), not actually providing any evidence that this form is *commonly* used in the sense of 'I ache' / 'I'm aching'. Although I cannot make any concrete claim about the actual statistical frequency of this English form, I wish to express my scepticism as to the plausibility of 'equating' it with the Greek intransitive personal form *ponao* / *ponas*. In other words, despite the fact that the functional analysis of *ponao* / *ponas* can be mapped onto that of *I hurt* / *I'm hurting* (see section 6.4 below), the very high frequency of the Greek form compared to the scarcity (or virtually, non-occurrence) of the English one, prevents us from suggesting that they are functionally equivalent in the construal of pain in everyday life.

tioning as a pain avowal approximating to the primitive cry (see the relevant discussion below), it is also the predominant form whereby the patient introduces himself as a suffering self before describing his painful condition, i.e. before attempting to identify and locate it. Thus, *ponao* is not only the most prevalent pain configuration used by patients as an expression of pain, i.e. an alternative to an interjection, a sigh, or a cry, it is also the most common form employed by pain sufferers as a means to set the stage for the subsequent description of their pain.

The statistical prevalence of *ponao* / *ponas* in the material of the present study is, in fact, quite striking as it represents almost half of all the collected data (47%), while the intransitive-impersonal *ponai*, which is the second most frequently observed form, covers one fifth of the constructions. Moreover, as we shall see in the detailed analysis of pain constructions (in terms of type of process and participant role(s) illustrated by relevant passages drawn from the corpus dialogues), like the intransitive-personal *ponao*, the intransitive-impersonal *ponai* in patients' speech can also be seen as often "replacing the primitive cry" in Wittgenstein's (1953/1989) sense. Hence, in patients' talk, alongside *ponao*, the form *ponai* reflects the expressive function of pain language in the sense that both *ponao* avowals and *ponai* utterances, especially when used on their own, can be interpreted as primarily functioning like interjections or cries of complaint rather than pain descriptions.

Another difference to note between patients' and doctors' data is that, though surprisingly quite infrequent, the transitive configuration *to xeri mu me ponai* 'my arm's hurting me' is four times more frequent in patients' material (9.53%) than it is in doctors' (2.44%). If we relate these figures to those of the other pain construal where the body part is expressed (or understood as a result of subject suppression), namely, the intransitive *to xeri mu ponai* 'my arm hurts' / 'my arm's hurting' (15.14% for patients and 14.25% for doctors), the picture that emerges is that, though overall quite infrequently expressed, the body part occurs more frequently in patients' verbalisations rather than in doctors'. In my understanding, this can be attributed to the fact that, when the patient is able to objectify his pain, he may identify its locus and quite naturally refer to it, while, on the other hand, the medical expert is actually concerned with locating the pain.

Overall, in the construal of pain as process, the body part is expressed or understood in only about one fifth of the constructions. Notably, in about 15% of the cases it is the grammatical subject of an intransitive structure, while in only 6% is it the subject of a two-participant construction whose syntactic object is the sufferer, e.g. *to xeri mu me ponai* 'my arm's hurting me'. Yet, as will be suggested in the relevant discussion of (22) below, in such constructions the two participants (body part and person) stand in a part-whole relationship and, therefore, the body part cannot be understood as a *distinct external* cause, i.e. as a separate entity causing pain to the sufferer as a whole. In other words, the sufferer is not understood as being 'split' into body part (aggressor) and self (sufferer). Rather, the body, where the self resides, is taken as a whole and it is pain which is seen as an external aggressor taking over both the afflicted body and the suffering self.

All this brings us to the relation between 'body' and 'self', which has been approached from various perspectives. A thorough examination of this issue, however, is beyond the scope of the present study. To highlight my account, I shall briefly mention just a few insightful views expressed by researchers working in different fields. In these analyses, the self may be perceived as either being contained within the body or as containing the body. Besides, the body may be identified as the self or it may be seen as an inseparable aspect of self.

Thus, according to the prevalent modern idea of a coherent and consistent self (e.g. Foucault, 1991, 1992; Gergen, 1991; Harre, 1991), the self is embodied, i.e. it is contained within the body, which provides boundaries that must be protected. Interestingly, though Melzack (1993) approaches the relation of 'body' and 'self' from a medical point of view, his remarks could be seen as actually converging with the more philosophical considerations expressed above. More specifically, according to him

> the body is perceived as a unity and is identified as the 'self', distinct from other people and the surrounding world. The experience of a unity of such diverse feelings including the self as the point of orientation in the surrounding environment, is produced by central neural processes [...] [which produce] a neurosignature pattern of a whole body.

Moreover, from the viewpoint of their health care professions, Paulson, Danielson and Söderberg (2002: 246) propose that the body is the medium through which conceptions of self are formed. "Body and self are inseparable but not identical; the body is an aspect of self, but in illness the experience of being-in-the world is ruptured by incapacity." Hence, illness influences the self in different ways. On the other hand, within his cognitive semantics approach, Lakoff (1996: 93, 102) argues that a person must be conceptualised as having two parts, the *Subject* and the *Self*. The Subject, which is the locus of consciousness and rationality, the centre of all subjective experience, "normally resides inside the other half of us – the Self. The Self includes at the very least our bodies, our emotions, and that part of us that acts in the world."

To conclude, my understanding of the relation between body and self with respect to pain is best captured in the view that, though not identical, they are inseparable, the self being contained within the body, which is an aspect of self. These concepts will concern us again when we analyse the metaphorical understanding of pain in *ponos* constructions (Chapter 8).

Let us now turn to Table 3 which presents an attempt at identifying pain configurations in terms of their construal of pain as a chronic vs. an acute condition.

Table 3 Chronic vs. acute pain configurations

	Pain configurations					
Pain expression	**Patients %**		**Doctors %**		**Total %**	
	Chron.	**Acute**	**Chron.**	**Acute**	**Chron.**	**Acute**
ponao / ponas (eδo)	48.79	51.21	52.36	47.64	**50.60**	**49.40**
ponai (eδo)	8.91	91.09	16.00	84.00	**11.93**	**88.07**
to xeri mu ponai	65.79	34.21	45.16	54.84	**56.52**	**43.48**
me ponai (eδo)	37.21	62.79	31.25	68.75	**35.59**	**64.41**
afto ponai	100.0		100.0	100.0	**100.0**	**100.0**
afto me ponai		100.0		100.0		**100.0**
to xeri mu me ponai		100.0				
Total	36.74	63.26	41.21	58.79	**38.71**	**61.29**

As was mentioned earlier, the absence of a simple present – 'present-in-present' morphological distinction in Greek makes it imperative to rely on the context in order to interpret present tense pain utterances in terms of time reference. Consequently, the distinction between chronic and acute pain can only be drawn on the basis of the context in which a pain pattern is actually uttered. Table 3 is the result of an attempt to assign, somewhat artificially perhaps, every single utterance either a chronic or an acute reading, with the hope that it might provide some indication as to how these forms are implemented in real life contexts.

It is not without reservations, however, that Table 3 should be interpreted, given that some 'technical' problems are involved. For example, the construction *to xeri mu ponai* with both its readings is not fully represented, as it was impossible to include the corresponding 63 subjectless patterns, which had not initially been distinguished into chronic vs. acute but, rather, they had been computed separately under one category. Despite this limitation, the figures in this table may quite reliably be interpreted as indicating that, within the particular contexts of our doctor-patient dialogues, pain as process is configured significantly more frequently as an acute sensation (61.29%) rather than a chronic one (38.71%). What is more, this difference is greater in patients' utterances (63.26% vs. 36.74%) compared to doctors' speech (58.79% vs. 41.21%).

The prevailing 'acute' representation of pain could, in part, be attributed to the situational context of the data collection: patients exposing their painful condition to a pain clinic expert or in the course of a treatment / medical session, will, naturally, present the sensation(s) they are experiencing on that occasion primarily, as well as describe conditions of a more general or chronic situation. In fact, their speech will normally alternate from the expression of their pain to the description of the general condition. Similarly, a medical expert, in the course of an interview or examination, will ask questions to collect information about the general state of the patient (e.g. when, how often, how intensely he suffers), but he will mostly focus on the patient's reactions and responses at the specific time, thus, resorting to constructions aimed at prompting the patient's verbalisation of the sensation(s) he is experiencing then and there. Besides, he may try to identify chronic pain on the basis of instances of pain deliberately induced to the patient at the time of the consultation, thus making the patient experience acute instances of his otherwise chronic painful condition.

The following extracts from the dialogues are meant to exemplify the difficulty of drawing the distinction between acute and chronic pain on the basis of pain verbalisations and the importance of the context in assigning a particular reading. Thus, while examples (1)-(2) and (3)-(4) seem to represent clear cases of chronic and acute pain, respectively, in (5) and (6) we observe a blending of the two readings in the verb forms printed in italics, as a result of which decision-making with respect to selecting a single interpretation is both difficult and arbitrary to a large extent. Yet, I suggest that wherever the context provides a clear indication of pain occurring on the spot (e.g. *stripse tora* 'turn now', *stasu, stasu, s'afti ti θesi* 'hold on, hold on, in this position') the corresponding forms can be interpreted as having a prevalent 'acute pain' reading, while the 'chronic pain' interpretation may be assigned to those forms that co-occur with clause constituents indicating duration, usual course of events or repetition (e.g. *tora enamisi xrono sinexja* 'now for the last one and a half years continuously', *otan arxizo na to sikono* 'when I start to lift it', *ama to voiθas etsi* 'when you help it like this'):

(1) P: tora enamisi xrono *ponao* sinexja…
now one-and-a-half year-ACC hurt-PRS:1SG continuously
'Now for the last one and a half year *I have been hurting* continuously…'

(2) D: pote *ponai* perisotero, otan milate, otan iste se iremia?
when hurt-PRS:3SG:IMPERS more when speak-PRS:2PL when be-PRS:2PL in quietness-ACC
'When *does it hurt* more, when you speak, when you are in a quiet state?'

(3) P: aaax! δen boro, θa me ksekanis! re si, *ponao*, to katalavenis?
ouch not can-PRS:1SG will I-ACC wear-out-PRS:2SG eh you-VOC hurt-PRS:1SG it-ACC understand-PRS:2SG
'Ouch! I can't take it, you will wear me out! Eh you, *I'm hurting*, don't you understand?'

(4) P: ax, kale, *ponai* poli, kale! kapu alu patas tora.
oh dear-VOC hurt-PRS:3SG:IMPERS a-lot dear-VOC somewhere else press-PRS:2SG now
'Oh dear, *it's hurting* a lot, dear! You're putting pressure somewhere else now.'

(5) D: sikose to pali. ti enjoses?
lift-IMP:2SG it-ACC again what-ACC feel-PST:2SG
'Lift it once more. What did you feel?'

P: otan arxizo na to sikono ponao. pono, otan pari afti ti θesi… eδo s'afti ti θesi *pono* poli. ke eδo *pono*.
when start-PRS:1SG to-PARTCL it-ACC lift-PRS:1SG hurt-PRS:1SG hurt-PRS:1SG when take-PRS:3SG this-ACC the position-ACC here in this-ACC the position-ACC hurt-PRS:1SG a-lot and here hurt-PRS:1SG
'When I start to lift it I hurt. I hurt when it takes this position… here in this position *I hurt / I'm hurting* a lot. Here, too, *I hurt / I'm hurting*.'

(6) D: […] ja stripse tora.
just turn-IMP:2SG now
'Just turn now.'

P: ponao!… eδo *ponai*. liγotero. ama to voiθas etsi δen ponai toso poli. *ponai*.
hurt-PRS:1SG here hurt-PRS:3SG:IMPERS less when it-ACC help-PRS:2SG like-this not hurt-PRS:3SG:IMPERS so much hurt-PRS:3SG:IMPERS
'I'm hurting!… *It hurts / It's hurting* here. Less. When you help it like this, it doesn't hurt so much. *It hurts / It's hurting*.'

D: *ponai*, e?
hurt-PRS:3SG:IMPERS eh
'*It hurts, does it*? / *It's hurting, is it*?'

P: eki, ne, ama pao pjo piso, ponai pjo…
there yes when go-PRS:1SG further back hurt-PRS:3SG:IMPERS more
'There, yes, when I move further back, it hurts more…'

D: stasu, stasu, s'afti ti θesi, min pas perisotero. pes mu an se *ponai* afto.
hold-on-IMP:2SG hold-on-IMP:2SG in this-ACC the position-ACC not go-IMP:2SG further tell-IMP:2SG I-GEN if you-ACC hurt-PRS:3SG this-NOM
'Hold on, hold on, in this position, don't move any further. Tell me if this *hurts / is hurting* you.'

Finally, I shall examine the total of the forms observed on the basis of two aspects, namely, their occurrence in transitive / intransitive constructions and their personal / impersonal character, to be further analysed and interpreted in the subsequent discussion.

Table 4 Transitive vs. intransitive pain constructions

Verb configurations				
Pain expression	**Type of structure**	**Pat %**	**Doc %**	**Total %**
ponao / ponas (eδo)? 'I hurt / I'm hurting (here)' 'do you hurt / are you hurting (here)?'	intransitive-personal	41.23	53.94	**46.82**
ponai (eδo) 'it hurts / it's hurting (here)'	intransitive-impersonal	20.12	19.08	**19.66**
to xeri mu (mu) ponai 'my arm hurts / my arm's hurting (in me)'	intransitive + body part	15.14	14.25	**14.75**
afto ponai 'that hurts'	intransitive-agentive (*afto* other than body part)	3.59	2.04	**2.90**
Total of intransitives		80.08	89.31	**84.13**
me ponai (eδo) 'it hurts me / it's hurting me (here)'	transitive-impersonal	8.57	4.07	**6.59**
to xeri mu me ponai 'my arm's hurting me'	transitive + body part	8.96	2.29	**6.03**
afto me ponai 'that's hurting me'	transitive (*afto* other than body part)	1.59	3.31	**2.35**
me ponas / se ponao? 'you're hurting me'/ 'am I hurting you?'	transitive-personal	0.80	1.02	**0.90**
Total of transitives		19.92	10.69	15.87
Grand total		100.0	100.0	**100.0**

Table 5 Personal vs. impersonal pain constructions

	Verb configurations			
Pain expression	**Type of structure**	**Pat %**	**Doc %**	**Total %**
ponao / **ponas (eδo)?** 'I hurt / I'm hurting (here)' 'do you hurt / are you hurting (here)?'	intransitive-personal	41.23	53.94	**46.82**
to xeri mu (mu) ponai 'my arm hurts / my arm's hurting (in me)'	intransitive + body part	15.14	14.25	**14.75**
to xeri mu me ponai 'my arm's hurting me'	transitive + body part	8.96	2.29	**6.03**
afto ponai 'that hurts'	intransitive-agentive (*afto* other than body part)	3.59	2.04	**2.90**
afto me ponai 'that's hurting me'	transitive (*afto* other than body part)	1.59	3.31	**2.35**
me ponas / **se ponao?** 'you're hurting me'/ 'am I hurting you?'	transitive-personal	0.80	1.02	**0.90**
Total of personal constructions		71.31	76.85	**73.74**
ponai (eδo) 'it hurts / it's hurting (here)'	intransitive-impersonal	20.12	19.08	**19.66**
me ponai (eδo) 'it hurts me / it's hurting me (here)'	transitive-impersonal	8.57	4.07	**6.59**
Total of impersonal constructions		28.69	23.15	**26.26**
Grand total		100.0	100.0	**100.0**

In Table 4, transitive and intransitive pain constructions have been listed and computed separately and appear in descending order of frequency. Thus, according to our data, in the overwhelming majority of Greek expressions (84.13%, i.e. 80.08% for patients and 89.31% for doctors), pain is construed as an intransitive process, e.g. *ponao / ponas (eδo), ponai (eδo), to xeri mu ponai*, and *afto ponai.*[5] Moreover, as we can see in Table 5, pain constructions are also predominantly 'personal' (73.74%) in both patients' and doctors' subcorpora (71.31% and 76.85%, respectively), e.g. *to xeri mu me ponai, ponao / ponas (eδo), to xeri mu ponai, afto ponai.*

If the figures of Tables 4 and 5 are juxtaposed, it will become clear that the majority of both personal (83.50%) and impersonal (74.89%) constructions are intransitive. Therefore, for the most part, pain structures are consistently, on the one hand, intransitive and, on the other, personal. Notably, of these two characteristics, it is the intransitive nature of pain expressions that is more prevalent. In actual fact, the extremely high frequencies of the constructions having the characteristic of intransitive and/or personal in the material of the present large-scale study not only reconfirm but also reinforce the claim first put forward in Lascaratou and Hatzidaki (2002) about the dual, i.e. intransitive-personal, character of pain configurations. Hence, now I can even more confidently claim that in Greek there is a clear tendency for pain to be primarily configured as an intransitive personal process.

To conclude this presentation of the general characteristics of pain as process in Greek, I am tempted to suggest that its predominantly intransitive character could further be elucidated if it were related to the findings of a number of psycholinguistic and neurolinguistic studies where it is argued that the acquisition and loss of verbs correlate with their argument structure properties leading to a superiority of intransitive verbs over transitives.

To be more specific, in De Bleser and Kauschke (2003), on the basis of data on verb processing elicited from (a) children acquiring German and (b) German aphasic adults, it is claimed that in both populations there is a clear tendency to prefer intransitive verbs over transitives, which supports the assumption of correspondence between the acquisition and breakdown of the ability to name verbs and their subcategories. In the group of children this preference is more noticeable in the early and late stages of acquisition. These findings constitute counter-evidence against Davidoff and Masterson's (1995) results, according to which English children were observed to name transitive verbs on a par with nouns and before intransitives. Moreover, De Bleser and Kauschke's data contradict the hypothesis put forward by Jonkers and Bastiaanse (1996, 1998), namely, that transitive verbs are easier than intransitives both for fluent and non-fluent aphasics. On the contrary, their findings show that in the majority of individual cases with agrammatic speech production there is a significant preference for intransitive verbs.

5. Our empirical data actually reflect Theophanopoulou-Kontou's (personal communication) observation that, *ponao* 'I hurt' is prototypically an intransitive verb denoting psychological state and, therefore, it more naturally occurs in intransitive ergative / unaccusative structures, its transitive causative patterns being somewhat secondary, e.g. *me ponas* 'you're hurting me' in the sense of *me kanis ke ponao* 'you make me hurt / suffer'.

The crucial point in De Bleser and Kauschke's (2003: 225–226) study that interests our analysis is the suggestion that this clear tendency to prefer intransitive verbs observed in children and aphasic adults can be accounted for in terms of the subcategories of verbs. They argue that their results for agrammatic aphasic patients conform to the claims expressed by Kim and Thompson (2000) and Thompson, Lange, Schneider, and Shapiro (1997), who suggest that the difficulty experienced by agrammatic patients in verb production tasks requiring conscious recall and self-generation of information reflects the argument structure of verbs. Thus, verbs with more arguments, e.g. transitives, display increased difficulty of lexical access compared to verbs with fewer arguments, e.g. intransitives. De Bleser and Kauschke argue that this interpretation of the superiority of intransitive verbs over transitives gains further support in their study, where it was found that intransitive verbs were not only generally acquired earlier than transitive ones, but were also more resistant to loss.

Drawing on the claims essentially put forward by these studies, it seems plausible to propose that, due to their simpler, more accessible argument structure properties, intransitive pain constructions represent a more direct form of expression compared to configurations constructing pain as a multi-argument process. In particular, intransitive first-person *ponao* and third-person impersonal *ponai* utterances lend themselves to voicing pain in the form of an automatic response. What is more, in Greek a considerable number of other physiological and psychological experiences are also primarily construed as intransitive processes. Consider such intransitive verbs as *pinao* 'I'm hungry', *δipsao* 'I'm thirsty', *nistazo* 'I feel sleepy', *fovame* 'I'm afraid' and *peθeno* 'I die' / 'I'm dying', whereby vital biological and mental processes are expressed. Alternatively, though less frequently, these processes can also be configured as *ime* + pseudo-participle relational attributive constructions: *ime pinazmenos* 'I'm hungry', *ime δipsazmenos* 'I'm thirsty', *ime nistaymenos* 'I'm sleepy', *ime fovizmenos* 'I'm afraid' and *ime peθamenos* 'I'm dead'.

6.4 Process types and structural functions in *ponao* constructions

Let us now look at each one of these pain expressions separately and see what they reveal to us about how Greek construes pain. In the present analysis, the constructions are discussed in descending order of frequency, which does not coincide with their order of presentation in Appendix A, where they are schematically presented, together with the corresponding English ones, as analysed along the lines of Halliday's paradigm. Wherever necessary, however, the Greek constructions will be referred to by means of their numbering in that paradigm. Our discussion is illustrated by representative examples drawn from the corpus.

(7) ***ponao* (*eδo*) /** Nos 3 & 3a of the paradigm
***ponas* (*eδo*)?** Nos 4 & 4a of the paradigm
hurt-PRS:1SG (here)
hurt-PRS:2SG (here)
'I hurt / I'm hurting (here)'
'do you hurt / are you hurting (here)?'

When *ponao* (*eδo*) corresponds to *I hurt* (*here*),[6] it is interpreted as relational: attributive, i.e. as a process whereby an entity *x*, the Carrier, is construed as having some quality *a*, the Attribute, ascribed to it. Thus, a relation is established between the Carrier and the Attribute.

This is, however, a very special case of relational attributive clause for two reasons. First, unlike typical attributive clauses where the Attribute is a distinct clause element realised as an NP, an AP or a PP, here the Attribute is conflated with the Process itself. Thus, pain as process is configured as some kind of quality attributed to the Carrier, despite the absence of such a typically distinct clause element. Secondly, and most importantly, it is the person rather than a body part which functions as the Carrier. Moreover, given that personal pronoun subjects are not expressed in Greek, unless emphatic or contrastive, the Carrier is linguistically realised through the verb suffix. As a consequence, the first-person *ponao* (No 3) and the second-person *ponas* (No 3a), mostly occurring in doctors' interrogative utterances, may form complete clauses on their own: the bare verb form realises simultaneously three components of the process, i.e. the Process itself, the Carrier, and the Attribute in conflation with the Process. Hence, it represents a very 'dense' construal of pain, one in which the experience of pain is represented as some kind of property of the sufferer, who, in turn, is not formally distinguishable from the Process / Attribute configuration. This is exemplified in the following extracts from our dialogues:[7]

(8) P: merikes fores *pono* ke arketa endona. merikes fores *pono* liγotero.
sometimes hurt-PRS:1SG and quite intensely sometimes hurt-PRS:1SG less
'Sometimes *I* even *hurt* quite intensely. Sometimes *I hurt* less.'
D: ine mera pu *δen ponate* kaθolu?
be-PRS:3SG day-NOM when not hurt-PRS:2PL at-all
'Is there any day when *you don't hurt* at all?'
P: iparxi ke… oxi, olokliri mera. orizmenes ores *δen pono*…
exist-PRS:3SG and no whole day-NOM some hours-ACC not hurt-PRS:1SG
'There is also… no, the whole day. For some hours *I don't hurt*…'

6. See note 4 above.

7. As was noted in Chapter 5, in the very few cases where a third-person, besides the patient and medical expert, takes part in the dialogue, I have used R (relative) to denote him/her.

(9) D: ne, pote *ponate* perisotero, otan iste ksaplomeni, otan iste kaθisti?
yes when hurt-PRS:2PL more when be-PRS:2PL lying-down when be-PRS:2PL seated
'Yes, when *do you hurt* more, when you are lying down or when you are seated?'

P: ksaploti otan ime ke otan perpatao *δen ponao* poli. otan im' akiniti, *ponao* poli, δen boro.
lying-down when be-PRS:1SG and when walk-PRS:1SG not hurt-PRS:1SG much when be-PRS:1SG still-NOM hurt-PRS:1SG much not can-PRS:1SG
'When I'm lying down and when I'm walking, *I don't hurt* a lot. When I don't move, *I hurt* a lot, I can't.'

(10) P: *ponao* ke tin imera.
hurt-PRS:1SG and the day-ACC
'*I hurt* during the day, too.'

R: *ponai, ponai.*
hurt-PRS:3SG hurt-PRS:3SG
'*He hurts, he hurts.*'

P: *ponao* ke tin imera, *ponao* ke tin imera ala kapu apasxolume ke ksexnieme, ala to vraδi ine to δrama, to vraδi ine to δrama.
hurt-PRS:1SG and the day-ACC hurt-PRS:1SG and the day-ACC but somehow keep-busy-PRS:1SG and forget-myself-PRS:1SG but the evening-ACC be-PRS:3SG the drama-NOM the evening-ACC be-PRS:3SG the drama-NOM
'*I hurt* in the daytime, too, *I hurt* in the daytime, too, but I keep myself busy somehow and I forget, but the tragedy is during the evening, the tragedy is during the evening.'

Though Halliday himself does not make this association, I shall further elaborate my analysis by comparing *I hurt* and the corresponding Greek *ponao* configurations to clauses expressing emotions such as *I'm glad / sorry / afraid / doubtful / upset / pleased / worried / sad / happy*, which Halliday analyses as a special variety of attributive clause. In these, he suggests, "the Attribute denotes a quality equivalent to a mental process, […] with Carrier equivalent to Senser" (1985/1994: 121). In such emotion clauses, however, the Attribute is not conflated with the Process, but rather, it 'corresponds' to a Process. Thus, on the one hand, *ponao* intransitive configurations, which represent almost half of the collected constructions of pain as process, and their corresponding English *I hurt* patterns are atypical relational attributive processes, in that the Attribute is conflated with the Process in a single form, i.e. that of a verb. On the other, we observe, English emotion clauses of the *I'm happy / worried* type are in a sense the obverse case, since they are structured like typical relational attributive clauses but the quality expressed by the Attribute in the form of an adjective (or pseudo-participle) is actually equivalent to a mental process, i.e. one normally realised as a verb.

This brings us back to Wierzbicka's analysis of the difference between Russian and English in the framing of emotions, the former favouring a verbal pattern and the latter an adjectival one. Wierzbicka's interpretation of this dissimilarity in constructing emotions may be usefully related to our finding that in the majority of Greek pain utterances the relation between the sufferer and his painful condition is established as an Attribute ascribed to him in the form of a processual verb, rather than as an adjectival or nominal complement.

Interestingly, there is a very subtle point in Wierzbicka's (1992: 401) account, that lends support to my intuitions about the essence of construing a sensation such as pain by means of verbs, and in particular, intransitive verbs. That is, Wierzbicka argues that it is by virtue of specific grammatical properties of verbs, such as their intransitive and reflexive nature, that the linguistic realisation of emotions as verbs in Russian reflects their understanding as inner activities and active, self-induced, processual events. (See also Pavlenko, 2002: 212–213)

On the other hand, Wierzbicka (1992: 400-401) relates the scarcity of the verbal pattern and the prevalence of the adjectival one in framing emotions in English to what she claims to be an important difference between these two patterns regarding the external manifestation of feelings: there is, she argues, a typical tendency for emotions designated by verbs of emotion – but not for those designated by adjectives of emotion – "to be expressed in action, often externally observable action. For example, a person who *rejoices* is probably doing something because of this feeling – dancing, singing, laughing, and so on." Yet, she points out, this inference is not spelt out as a certainty and, therefore, it would be safer to treat the dynamic character of such verbs more cautiously. Wierzbicka's assumption that the verbal pattern in construction of emotions tends to have an actional, dynamic, and public dimension largely underlies her cultural interpretation of the increasing infrequency of English intransitive verbs of emotion, e.g. *grieve*, *worry* or *pine*.[8] In her view, this infrequency may be understood in terms of the socio-cultural Anglo-Saxon attitude whereby people are expected to control their emotions and refrain from externally observable emotional manifestations: 'emotional' behaviour tends to be treated with disapproval, suspicion and embarrassment. People are, therefore, encouraged "to be *glad* rather than to *rejoice*, to be *sad* rather than to *pine*, to be *angry* rather than to *fume* or *rage*, and so on" (*ibid.*: 401). Hence, there is a tendency for

8. According to Wierzbicka (1992: 401), not only does the category of English intransitive verbs of emotion comprise very few members, e.g. *worry*, *grieve*, *rejoice*, *pine*, etc., but also the category as a whole may be losing ground in the modern language.

English intransitive emotion verbs, e.g. *sulk*, *fret*, *fume*, *rave*, to be understood as expressing "negative disappointing tones." (See also Wierzbicka, 1988: 253–254.)

Without actually adopting Wierzbicka's cross-linguistic and cross-cultural analysis of the framing of emotions, I suggest that her cultural interpretation of the framing of emotions in English may indirectly shed light on the analysis of the reverse situation prevailing in Greek pain constructions. In other words, it seems to me that we may be able to reach a better understanding if, in relating and extending Halliday's functional account of English emotion clauses to the study of Greek pain configurations, Wierzbicka's insights with respect to the verbal vs. the adjectival framing of emotions are also taken into account. Hence, the image that emerges is that Greek does not favour the construal of pain in the guise of typical relational attributive clauses structured with an adjective (or pseudo-participle), but rather its representation by means of verbs reflecting its processual aspect, very much like Russian and unlike English in the construction of emotions. Moreover, I suggest that a culturally based study of the language of pain in Greek might reveal an underlying cultural factor encouraging Greek speakers to use *ponao* 'to hurt' rather than ??*ime ponemenos* 'to be sore', thus resorting to more dynamic, social, and processual framings of pain.[9]

9. It is worth noting here an interesting point made by Pavlenko (2002: 226) as regards emotion construction in Russian, which indirectly links emotion words with the processes of feeling, suffering, and pain. Thus, she draws our attention to "the social character of emotions whereby people can be engaged in the process of co-feeling, as expressed in the verbs *sochuvstvovat'* 'to sympathize' (literally: to co-feel) and *soperezhivat'* 'to empathize' (literally: to co-suffer things through), neither of which has exact counterparts in American English." Just as in Russian, there exist in Greek a number of expressions agnate to the relational attributive construal of *ponao*, i.e. verbs expressing co-feeling: cf. *sinesθanome* 'I feel' / 'I'm conscious of' (*sin-esθanome*, literally: 'I co-feel'), *simbasxo* 'I suffer along with' (*sin-pasxo*, literally: 'I co-suffer'), and *simbono* 'I sympathise with', in the sense of *ime simbonetikos* 'I am compassionate' / 'I feel compassion for' (*sin-pono*, literally: 'I co-hurt'), all of which have derivative forms reinforcing this social aspect, e.g. *sinesθima* 'feeling' / 'sentiment', *simbaθia* 'liking' / 'sympathy', *simbonia* 'compassion', *simbonetikos* 'compassionate'. Hence, within a culturally based account of pain language it might be possible to argue, along the lines of Pavlenko, that the understanding of a dynamic and social framing of pain in Greek is reinforced by the existence of such verbs. Moreover, it should be noted that, unlike the *ime* + pseudo-participle periphrastic relational attributive constructions *ime pinazmenos*, *ime δipsazmenos*, *ime nistaymenos*, *ime fovizmenos*, and *ime peθamenos*, corresponding to the intransitive verbs *pinao* 'I'm hungry', *δipsao* 'I'm thirsty', *nistazo* 'I feel sleepy', *fovame* 'I'm afraid', and *peθeno* 'I die / I'm dying', the pattern *ime ponemenos* is quite marginally used to refer to bodily pain, while in the context of psychological suffering it occurs more naturally, e.g. *afti i jineka ine poli ponemeni* 'this woman has suffered a lot of pain'. On the other hand, the pseudo-participle *ponemenos* freely occurs as an Epithet, i.e. a modifier, e.g. *afto ine to ponemeno xeri* 'this is the painful arm', *i eleni ine ponemenos anθropos* 'Helen is a person who has suffered a lot of pain', the context of mental pain favouring its use.

As far as further interpretations of *ponao* constructions, there could be a possible secondary understanding as a behavioural process, agnate to mental: emotive clauses (cf. *anisixo* (*sti skepsi oti…*) 'I worry (at the thought that…)'), where the person would be assigned the Behaver function.

Moving on to *ponao* in the sense of 'I'm hurting' (Nos 4 and 4a), it can be interpreted as a material process, one of 'doing', which is typically more focused in time, having a clear beginning and ending. It is not, however, a process of 'doing something to anyone or anything' (Halliday, 1998: 19), as only one participant, the Actor, is involved. The process not being extended to another entity, in transitivity terms such a clause is intransitive, while in terms of voice the clause is middle and its single participant, i.e. the person, is the Actor / Medium. Hence, pain is configured as a process of 'doing' something which is carried out by the sufferer himself without being extended to another entity – a Goal – and without being caused by any, explicit or implicit, external Agent. Therefore, the painful experience is structured as self-engendering, though in actual fact, there must be an external agency involved. When uttered by the sufferer, such a clause is a pain avowal, a statement whereby he wishes to publicly declare that at the specific moment he is suffering as a whole, all by himself as if he were involved in a solitary action where there is no room for any other participant: just the sufferer – Actor / Medium – and his pain – the Process. That such avowals may have an exclamatory function and, hence, approximate to interjections, i.e. the most expressive linguistic signs (sitting next to automatic, natural reactions like cries / groans / screams) on the expressive-descriptive axis of our proposed continuum is further corroborated by the observation that in the data they often co-occur or alternate with typical pain exclamations, such as *axa! / ax! / a! / u! / ox! / oxu!* 'ah!' / 'oh!' / 'ouch!' or other interjections, e.g. *panajitsa mu* 'my (little / dear) Virgin Mary' (for example, (11), (12), (13), and (15) below). Clauses expressing other bodily processes, such as *emorayo* 'I'm bleeding', *psixorayo* 'I'm dying', are the closest agnates of *ponao* in the sense of 'I'm hurting'.

(11) P: *ponao,* xriso mu peδi. ax! ax panajitsa mu!
hurt-PRS:1SG golden my child-VOC ouch ouch Virgin-Mary-DIMIN:VOC my
'*I'm hurting*, my sweet child. Ouch! Ouch, my (little / dear) Virgin Mary!'

D: (laughs)

P: mi jelas. ax! δen iparxi simio pu na min *ponao*… δeksia, δen boro na akumbiso kaθolu ute stin karekla.
not laugh-PRS:2SG ouch not exist-PRS:3SG point-NOM where to-PARTCL not hurt-PRS:1SG right not can-PRS:1SG to-PARTCL lean-PRS:1SG at-all nor on-the chair-ACC
'Don't laugh. Ouch! There is no part (of my body) where *I'm not hurting*… On the right, I can't even lean on the chair.'

(12) D: eδo?
here
'Here?'

P: *ponao*, min sproxnis poli.
hurt-PRS:1SG, not push-IMP:2SG much
'*I'm hurting*, don't push too hard.'

D: eδo *ponas*? eδo perissotero?
here hurt-PRS:2SG here more
'*Are you hurting* here? Here more?'

P: oxu! oxu! oxu! eki, eki!
ouch ouch ouch there there
'Ouch! Ouch! Ouch! There, there!'

D: eδo?
here
'Here?'

P: oxi, eki.
not there
'No, there.'

D: eδo?
here
'Here?'

P: *ponao*! ox! ox! ox! ox! ox! ox! ox! ox! ox! ox! ox! ine poli… poli *ponao*!
hurt-PRS:1SG oh oh oh oh oh oh oh oh oh oh oh be-PRS:3SG very much hurt-PRS:1SG
'*I'm hurting*! Oh! Oh! Oh! Oh! Oh! Oh! Oh! Oh! Oh! Oh! Oh! It is very… *I'm hurting* a lot!'

(13) P: aaa! otan t' aplono, molis…
ouch when it-ACC stretch-PRS:1SG as-soon-as
'Ouch! When I stretch it, as soon as…'

D: *ponate*?
hurt-PRS:2PL
'*Are you hurting*?'

P: ne *ponao*.
yes hurt-PRS:1SG
'Yes, *I'm hurting*.'

D: tendoste, tendoste, oso borite, oso borite. δen borite alo?
stretch-IMP:2PL stretch-IMP:2PL as-much-as can-PRS:2PL as-much-as can-PRS:2PL not can-PRS:2PL anymore

'Stretch it, stretch it, as much as you can, as much as you can. Is that all you can do?'

P: na to tendoso akoma?
to-PARTCL it-ACC stretch-PFV:NON-PST:1SG more
'Shall I stretch it even more?'

D: ki alo de, exi akoma eδo poli...
and more come-on exist-PRS:3SG:IMPERS more here much
'Some more, come on, you can stretch it much more here...'

P: u! *ponao* poli.
ouch hurt-PRS:1SG a-lot
'Ouch! *I'm hurting* a lot.'

The strong preference, in terms of frequency of occurrence, for *ponao* 'I hurt' / 'I'm hurting' constructions cannot fully be accounted for only by reference to their experiential grammar but rather the textual component of grammar must also be invoked. I assume that in Greek, like in English and many other languages, the constituent that is placed in the clause initial position functions as the Theme of the utterance, i.e. it sets the scene, it provides the perspective for the presentation of the action or event to be communicated (Halliday, 1985/94, Ch.5; Fries, 1981/1983, 1992, 1995; Hasan and Fries, eds, 1995; Ghadessy, ed., 1995; Matthiessen, 1995a). In languages with a rigid Subject Verb Object (SVO) order, such as English, it follows that in declarative clauses the unmarked Theme is the syntactic Subject. However, this is not always the case in Greek, where, due to its word order flexibility, the Subject may end up in another position of the clause, despite the fact that in frequency terms SVO is the dominant order, to the effect that Greek is usually classified as an SVO language. (For this controversial issue, see Drachman, 1985; Greenberg, 1963/1966; Horrocks, 1983; Lascaratou, 1984, 1989, 1998; Philippaki-Warburton, 1985, 1987; Tsimpli, 1990; Tzartzanos, 1963, among others.) What is more, if the Subject is a personal pronoun rather than a lexical NP then it is suppressed, unless emphatic or contrastive. It follows, therefore, that in unmarked clauses the Subject of first and second-person verbs is not realised as a separate clause element. This, however, does not mean that it is completely absent, since subjectless Greek verbs actually 'incorporate' the subject *via* the personal ending, which is assumed to function as a reduced subject (see Philippaki-Warburton, 1987, 1992). Consequently, despite the absence of a pronoun in the form of a distinct constituent, i.e. *eγo* 'I', the first-person perspective is clearly mapped onto *ponao* utterances. Hence, it may be argued that in such construals of pain it is the sufferer as a whole, rather than some body part, that is presented as the setting of the painful experience, in much the same way as in those English clauses where the unmarked thematic position is occupied by the Subject *I*, e.g. *I hurt*, *I'm hurt-*

ing, I have a headache. "Where I start from, what I feel to be the setting of this unpleasant experience, is not my head, it is me – my self, as a whole", Halliday (1998: 4) argues.

The following two extracts from our doctor-patient dialogues are representative examples of the holistic construal of pain associated with *ponao* avowals:

(14) P: na, eδo, *olo mu to soma, olo to…*
right here whole-NOM my the body-NOM whole the-NOM
'Look, here, *my whole body, all the…*'
R: ne, pes esi stin kopela.
yes, say-IMP:2SG you-NOM to-the girl-ACC
'Yes, you tell the girl.'
P: *ponao*!
hurt-PRS:1SG
'*I hurt*!'
D: to soma olo i to poδi?
the body-NOM whole-NOM or the leg-NOM
'The whole body or (just) the leg?'
P: *ke to soma ke to poδi ke…*
and the body-NOM and the leg-NOM and
'*Not only the body (in general) but also the leg and…*'
R: ke ta nefra tis ke ola tis.
and the kidneys-NOM her and everything-NOM her
'As well as her kidneys and every part of her.'
P: ke *ola mu.*
and everything-NOM my
'And *every part of me.*'
D: apo pote ponate etsi?
since when hurt-PRS:2PL like-this
'Since when have you been hurting like this?'
P: mmm…
mmm
'Hmm…'
D: poli kero?
much time-ACC?
'For a long time?'
P: *ponao*!
hurt-PRS:1SG
'*I hurt*!'

(15) P: δen andexo, aaa!
not tolerate-PRS:1SG aaah
'I can't take it, aaah!'
D: ti δen andexis, na kunas to poδi i na'se 'δo mesa?
what not tolerate-PRS:2SG to-PARTCL move-PRS:2SG the leg-ACC or to-PARTCL be-PRS:2SG here inside
'What is it that you can't cope with, to move your leg or to be in here?'
P: *ponao*!
hurt-PRS:1SG
'*I'm hurting*!'
D: pu, more, ponas?
where dear hurt-PRS:2SG
'Where are you hurting, dear?'
P: *ponao*!
hurt-PRS:1SG
'*I'm hurting*!'
D: pu? pu? δikse mu pu ponas.
where where show-IMP:2SG I-GEN where hurt-PRS:2SG
'Where? Where? Show me where you are hurting.'
P: *olo*.
all-over
'*All over*.'

Summing up, I suggest that *ponao* utterances are very 'intense' pain avowals for two reasons: first, as regards their experiential grammar, they construe pain either as a relational process with the Attribute in conflation with the Process, or as a self-engendering material effective process, both construals bringing out the processual dimension of pain very vividly. Secondly, in terms of textual grammar, the sufferer's self is presented as part of the process *via* the verb suffix, thus providing a holistic thematic perspective for the communication of the unpleasant experience. In that respect, the intransitive *ponao* construction could also be related to the Greek passive, which has been argued by Lascaratou (1984) to be a device that "allows a transitive verb to be 'stripped' of its NP's and carry all the communicative dynamism by itself", given that about 90% of passive occurrences are agentless and Greek is a language suppressing personal pronoun subjects. Like the passive verb, which can form a full clause all by itself, i.e. a clause consisting of a rhematic verb alone with no theme realised as a distinct constituent, I suggest that *ponao* expresses the most rhematic encoding of the pain experience.[10]

Finally, a secondary interpretation of *ponao* could be behavioural, a process of typically human physiological and psychological behaviour, with the person as Behaver (cf. *tremo* 'I'm trembling'). Besides, there could be a further interpretation as existential: occurring, with the Medium, i.e. the person, functioning as a kind of Setting (cf. *kriono* 'I'm feeling cold'), where pain is understood to exist, to occur. I suggest that this is a special type of existential process since, in my understanding, the Existent, which is typically the Medium in existential clauses, seems to be conflated here with the Process, and the function of Medium is taken up by the person, thus providing a setting for pain to occur, to dwell. This secondary existential understanding of *ponao* relates it to the impersonal *ponai* 'it hurts' / 'it's hurting', which is the next most frequently observed configuration in the data, having an exclusively existential interpretation.

(16) ***ponai* (*eδo*)** Nos 5 & 6 of the paradigm
hurt-PRS:3SG:IMPERS (here)
'it hurts / it's hurting (here)'

Once more, the Greek pattern corresponds to two English ones, that is *it hurts* (*here*) and *it's hurting* (*here*) (Nos 5 and 6 of the paradigm, respectively).

In the first case, the third-person singular suffix, incorporated in the verb form *ponai*, functions as an impersonal Setting, like *it* in *it hurts*, the plural *ponane* 'they hurt' not being a possible variant, in the same way that *they* cannot replace *it* in English. Pain is interpreted as an existential process of the 'existing' type, one located on the borderline between material and relational processes, a process in which something is simply represented as existing. Thus, according to this interpretation, *ponai* (*eδo*) is understood as 'there is / there exists (a) pain (here)'. When used by the patient, therefore, it serves the purpose of basically communicating his awareness that there exists pain either in a specific locus identified by a locative adverbial, e.g. *eδo* 'here', *eki* 'there', or in an unspecified location construed as an impersonal Setting (cf. *γlistrai eδo* 'it's slippery here', *vromai eδo* 'it stinks here', i.e. *iparxi kapja δisosmia eδo* 'there is a stink here'). Consider the following dialogue where in response to the doctor's question about the duration of pain, the condi-

10. According to the analysis of *ponao* as a primarily unaccusative verb, presented in note 5 above, there is a difference between such agentless passive constructions as *katastrafika* 'I got / am destroyed', and intransitive *ponao* avowals. The difference concerns the possibility or not of an agentive interpretation. In the case of *katastrafika* this possibility exists, since there is an ambiguity between a reflexive reading (*apo mena* 'by myself') and a clearly passive agentive one (*apo kapjon* 'by someone'). With *ponao*, however, only an internal Cause is possible, external Agents being excluded from unaccusative patterns.

tions under which it becomes more intense, and its location, the patient consistently uses the impersonal *ponai* to state the existence of his pain:

(17) D: θelo na mu pis, ine sinexomenos o ponos, *ponai* sinexja?
want-PRS:1SG to-PARTCL I-GEN tell-PFV:NON-PST:2SG be-PRS:3SG continuous the pain-NOM hurt-PRS:3SG:IMPERS continuously
'I want you to tell me, is the pain continuous, *does it hurt* continuously?'

P: ne.
yes
'Yes.'

D: ja periγrapse ton. pote *ponai* perisotero, otan ise ksapla, otan ise orθios, otan perpatas, pote, otan kaθese?
just describe-IMP:2SG it-ACC when hurt-PRS:3SG:IMPERS more when be-PRS:2SG lying-down when be-PRS:2SG standing when walk-PRS:2SG when when sit-PRS:2SG
'Just describe it. When *does it hurt* more, when you're lying down, when you're standing, when you're walking, when, when you're sitting?'

P: otan kaθome parapano *ponai*, ksaplomenos me ponai, perpatao eee ma *ponai*, ma kalitera, pernai… otan perpatao.
when sit-PRS:1SG more hurt-PRS:3SG:IMPERS lying-down I-ACC hurt-PRS:3SG:IMPERS walk-PRS:1SG eh but hurt-PRS:3SG:IMPERS but better go-away-PRS:3SG:IMPERS when walk-PRS:1SG
'When I sit longer, *it hurts*, when I'm lying down it hurts me, I walk, eh, sometimes *it hurts*, other times it's better, it goes away… when I walk.'

D: otan perpatas ine kaliteros, *ponai* liγotero.
when walk-PRS:2SG be-PRS:3SG better-NOM hurt-PRS:3SG: IMPERS less
'When you walk, it's better, *it hurts* less.'

P: ne.
yes
'Yes.'

D: eno ksapla?
whereas lying-down
'Whereas when lying down?'

P: *ponai.*
hurt-PRS:3SG:IMPERS
'*It hurts.*'

D: *ponai.*
hurt-PRS:3SG:IMPERS
'*It hurts.*'

When *ponai* (*eδo*) is equivalent to *it's hurting* (*here*), it is configured as an existential process of the 'occurring' type. By placing such existential processes closer to material ones, Halliday (1985/1994: 143–144) makes it possible to map them onto meteorological processes of the type *it's raining / hailing / snowing / freezing / pouring / drizzling / lightning / thundering*, which are a special category located between existential and material processes.

Among meteorological processes, such clauses as *vrexi* 'it's raining', *xionizi* 'it's snowing', *fisai* 'it's windy' *astrafti* 'it's lightning' are analysed as consisting only of a single element, i.e. the Process, or, to be more accurate, as having the obligatory element Medium conflated with the Process. On the analogy of such meteorological clauses, *ponai* in the sense of 'it's hurting' can be understood as consisting of a Process in conflation with the Medium. The understanding of such processes as consisting essentially of a single element, the Process itself, makes the construal of pain more dynamic, more actional, in the sense that its processual aspect is reinforced. This functional account provides an insightful interpretation of the everyday experience of pain as a phenomenon overtaking the sufferer, often without previous notice, something like an unexpected rain or, even worse, a sudden storm (cf. *vrexi* 'it's raining', *xionizi* 'it's snowing', *fisai* 'it's windy'). Thus, it captures the sufferer's feeling that pain 'happens' to him as if brought about by unspecified and/or indistinguishable factors, much the same as, at least for non weather-experts, drastic changes of the weather seem to occur as a result of uncontrollable natural forces. In Halliday's words (1998: 20), it is "as if the pain was a kind of weather going on inside the body." Seen from this perspective, the impersonal *ponai* is a pain configuration whereby the patient complains at a specific moment that he is being 'inflicted' by an unpleasant sensation, which simply 'happens' to him, thus, prompting his immediate reaction in the form of a cry of complaint. As in the case of *ponao*, my claim about the expressive function of *ponai* is highlighted by its frequent co-occurrence with characteristic pain exclamations, such as *ax! / a! / u! / au! / o! / mmm!* 'ah!' / 'oh!' / 'ouch!' / 'mmm!', e.g. (18)-(20) below. What is more, examining dialogues (18) and (19) we observe in two instances that, when asked by the medical expert to say what his pain is like, the patient, instead of providing a description of his sensation, simply expresses it by means of *ponai*. Hence, I assume this use of *ponai* as a spontaneous reaction to be an indication of its function as an exclamation or a comment, whereby the construal of pain as process is intensely brought out.

(18) P: a!
ouch
'Ouch!'

D: ti?
what
'What?'

P: a! a!
ouch ouch
'Ouch! Ouch!'

D: *ponai*?
hurt-PRS:3SG:IMPERS
'*Is it hurting*?'

P: ne.
yes
'Yes.'

D: pu *ponai*?
where hurt-PRS:3SG:IMPERS
'Where *is it hurting*?'

P: eki.
there
'There.'

D: eki? monon eki *ponai*? δen *ponai* puθena alu?
there only there hurt-PRS:3SG:IMPERS not hurt-PRS:3SG:IMPERS anywhere else
'There? *Is it hurting* only there? *Isn't it hurting* anywhere else?'

P: mono.
only
'Only.'

D: mono? pos ine aftos o ponos? ja pes mu.
only how be-PRS:3SG this the pain-NOM just tell-IMP:2SG I-GEN
'Only? How is this pain? Come on, tell me.'

P: *ponai*.
hurt-PRS:3SG:IMPERS
'*It's hurting*.'

(19) P: eki oxi. ax! ax! ax! *ponai* liγo. se orizmena simia.
there no ouch ouch ouch hurt-PRS:3SG:IMPERS a-bit at some points-ACC
'There no. Ouch! Ouch! Ouch! *It's hurting* a bit. At some points.'

D: se orizmena *ponai* pjo poli apo ala?
at some hurt-PRS:3SG:IMPERS more than others
'Is *it hurting* more at some (points) rather than at others?'

P: ne, ne, ne, afto afto eki me ponai para poli. ax! ax!
yes yes yes this this there I-ACC hurt-PRS:3SG:IMPERS very much ouch ouch
'Yes, yes, yes, that's hurting me a lot. Ouch! Ouch!'

D: pos ine?
how be-PRS:3SG
'What is it like?'

P: *ponai.*
hurt-PRS:3SG:IMPERS
'*It's hurting.*'

D: to iδjo?
the same
'The same?'

P: oxi, liγotero tora eki.
no less now there
'No, less there now.'

D: ti sas kani?
what you-ACC do-PRS:3SG:IMPERS
'What does it do to you?'

P: *ponai* ala oxi para poli.
hurt-PRS:3SG:IMPERS but not very much
'*It's hurting* but not that much.'

(20) D: ine ke o mis, ala prepi na ine ke i arθrosi. ja jirna… i arθrosi.
be-PRS:3SG and the muscle-NOM but must-PRS to-PARTCL be-PRS:3SG and the joint-NOM just turn-around-IMP:2SG the joint-NOM
'It's also the muscle, but it must be the joint too. Just turn around… the joint.'

P: a! *ponai.* aman! 29 ores! ores anamonis sto amsterdam… pjo poli eδo.
ouch hurt-PRS:3SG:IMPERS my-goodness 29 hours hours of-waiting in-the Amsterdam more here
'Ouch! *It's hurting.* My goodness! 29 hours! Hours waiting in Amsterdam… more here.'

D: ne, ne, pjo poli… stasu na δo. xalarose.
yes yes more stay-IMP:2SG to-PARTCL see-PFV:NON-PST:1SG relax-IMP:2SG
'Yes, yes, even more… let me see. Relax.'

P: mmm! o! aau, aau, aau! au!
mmm ouch ouch ouch ouch
'Mmm! Ouch! Ouch, ouch, ouch, ouch!'

(21) ***to xeri mu (mu) ponai*** Nos 1, 2, (1+2)a, & (1+2)b of the paradigm
the arm-NOM my (I-GEN) hurt-PRS:3SG
'my arm hurts / is hurting (in me)'

The expression *to xeri mu ponai* corresponds to *my arm hurts* and *my arm's hurting* (Nos 1 and 2, respectively).[11] Unlike *ponao* and *ponai*, in which the subject is typically realised by the verb suffix, here it is the part of the body which is the active Subject.

On the analogy of *ponao* 'I hurt', when *to xeri mu ponai* relates to *my arm hurts*, it is primarily construed as relational: attributive with the Process in conflation with the Attribute (cf. *i mustarδa kei* (*ine kafteri*) 'the mustard is hot', *i alifi kolai* (*ine koloδis*) 'the ointment is sticky'). In this construal, pain as process is once more understood as a quality attributed to the Carrier, which, unlike what happens in the case of *ponao*, is present in the form of a distinct clause element denoting the body part and functioning as a kind of Setting. In other words, by means of *to xeri mu ponai*, the sufferer identifies the part of his body that is painful by configuring it as the Carrier of the pain experience or quality. Hence, the locus of pain is specified as a part of the sufferer's body rather than as the sufferer's self configured holistically, which is the case in *ponao* 'I hurt'.

(22) P: ala *to kokalo eδo ponai*, ine enas staθeros ponos.
but the bone-NOM here hurt-PRS:3SG be-PRS:3SG a constant-NOM pain-NOM
'But *the bone hurts* here, it's a constant pain.'

(23) P: *ponan ta poδia mu* ke muδiazune.
hurt-PRS:3PL the legs-NOM my and get-numbed-PRS:3PL
'*My legs hurt* and get numbed.'

In the first of the following two extracts from the data we observe that the doctor uses the holistic configuration *ponate*? (second-person plural) to inquire about the patient's condition, the latter responding *ponai to poδi mu* 'my leg hurts', thus directly identifying the location of his pain. In the second example the patient himself initially presents his painful state holistically and then specifies the suffering part of his body.

(24) D: lipon, ja pite poso xronon iste?
well just tell-IMP:2PL how-many years-GEN be-PRS:2PL
'Well, just tell me how old are you?'

11. The category under (1+2)a represents the collected instances of structures 1 and 2 with suppressed subjects. In addition, category (1+2)b comprises the variations of structures 1 and 2 containing the malefactive genitive personal pronoun *mu* 'in me' which were only very marginally observed in our dialogues.

P: poso xronon ime?
how-many years-GEN be-PRS:1SG
'How old am I?'

D: ne.
yes
'Yes.'

P: exinda.
sixty
'Sixty.'

D: ke ponate?
and hurt-PRS:2PL
'And you hurt?'

P: *ponai to poδi mu.*
hurt-PRS:3SG the leg-NOM my
'My leg hurts.'

(25) P: jenika ime katavevlimeni. δen exo oreksi na fao, ponao, *ponai i plati mu i δeksia…*
generally be-PRS:1SG worn-out-NOM not have-PRS:1SG appetite-ACC to-PARTCL eat-PFV:NON-PST:1SG hurt-PRS:1SG hurt-PRS:3SG the back-NOM my the right-NOM
'I'm generally worn-out. I don't feel like eating, I hurt, *my back hurts on the right…'*

D: mmm
uhuh
'Uhuh.'

P: ee exo ponus δiaxitus.
eh eh have-PRS:1SG pains diffused-ACC
'Eh, I have pains all over my body.'

When it corresponds to *my arm's hurting*, the pattern *to xeri mu ponai*, like *ponao* 'I'm hurting', is interpreted as material: middle process with the body part as Actor / Medium (cf. *to xeri mu tremi* 'my hand's shaking'). This process, therefore, like *ponao*, is understood as one of 'doing', with a clear beginning and ending, but again the 'doing' is not extended to anyone or anything else, i.e. the clause is intransitive. Moreover, here it is the body part which is treated like the 'doer' of the deed rather than the sufferer himself. Besides, pain is construed as a self-engendering process, since no external Agent is explicitly or implicitly configured, although an external agency is definitely involved.

(26) P: oxu, mana mu!
ouch mother-VOC my
'Oh, mother!'
D: ti, kale, ti epaθes?
what dear what happen-to-you-PST:3SG
'What is it, dear, what happened to you?'
P: *ponai o γofos.*
hurt-PRS:3SG the hip
'*My hip's hurting.*'

To conclude, *to xeri mu ponai* in the sense of 'my arm's hurting', does not represent pain as a holistic experience in the way that *ponao* 'I'm hurting' does. Here, the sufferer does not simply avow his pain, he makes a step further: he locates it by construing a particular body part as the 'doer', the Actor of the 'doing'. By presenting his unfortunate condition as a more localised experience, he is able to gain some distance from it.

In a secondary interpretation, the Medium, that is the body part, acquires the function of Setting in a relational process of the existential: occurring type (cf. *to tavani stazi* 'the roof's leaking'). Thus, pain is interpreted as existing, as 'occurring' in the body part, which is not the 'doer' anymore, but rather the setting where pain resides.

(27) P: *to poδi mu… to δeksi… ponai…* ke mexri epano eki mexri to γonato.
the leg-NOM my the right-NOM hurt-PRS:3SG and as-high-as up there as-high-as the knee-ACC
'*My leg… the right one… is* even *hurting…* as high as there, as high as the knee.'

In this secondary reading, the pattern *to xeri mu ponai* means, more or less, 'there occurs pain in my arm', 'pain is occurring in my arm'. Therefore, such pain construals should be positioned further from the clearly expressive pole of the proposed continuum.

(28) ***to xeri mu me ponai*** Nos 7 & 7a of the paradigm
the arm-NOM my I-ACC hurt-PRS:3SG
'my arm's hurting me'

The expression *to xeri mu me ponai* is the equivalent of *my arm's hurting me*. Of all collected expressions with considerable frequencies, this is the least frequent one (6.03%), its salient feature being that it is the only one in which pain is construed as a process involving two participants, namely the body part and the person, the former affecting the latter, its owner.

This type of process is interpreted as belonging to mental: impacting processes which share properties of two types of process, namely, mental and material ones. In particular, mental impacting processes, by virtue of being processes of 'doing something mental to', are related to material processes which are processes of 'doing' *par excellence*. As a consequence, like material processes, they can be interpreted both as not clearly bounded in time and as having clear beginnings and endings. The exploration of the observed instances of this Greek construction type suggested that the process is chiefly represented as being more focused in time.[12]

On the other hand, despite the presence of two participants, no typical 'extension' of a 'doing' is involved here – as in the case of material: effective processes, e.g. *i yata mu me kiniyai* 'my cat is chasing me'. Therefore, the two participants cannot be assigned the functions of Actor and Goal which are characteristic of material processes but, rather, they represent the two distinctive participants of mental processes, i.e. Phenomenon and Senser. Thus, the body part and the self are mapped onto the transitive functions of Phenomenon (that which is 'sensed') and Senser (the being that is always 'endowed' with consciousness), respectively. Furthermore, in ergative terms, the body part, in addition to being the Phenomenon, is also the Agent, since the condition that the process be encoded in the direction from Phenomenon (subject) to Senser is met in this process type (Halliday, 1985/1994: 165).[13] (For a discussion of the subtle distinction between the transitive function Actor and the ergative function Agent, see Chapter 4, section 4.2.) Yet, what makes the semantics of this type of construction peculiar is that the two participants stand in a part-whole relationship: the Phenomenon is a body part of the self-Senser. Hence, despite its agentive interpretation, the Phenomenon part of the

12. Halliday (1998: 20) remarks that in English the mental: impacting processes of 'pain' "seem to be always present-in-present."

13. As was mentioned in Chapter 4, section 4.2, one of the distinctive features of mental processes is their bidirectionality in language, i.e. the possibility of representing them as two-way processes, namely, with the subject functioning as either the Senser or the Phenomenon, still keeping the clause in the active voice, e.g. *apolamvano to proino kafeδaki mu* 'I enjoy my morning (little) cup of coffee' or *to proino kafeδaki mu me efxaristi* 'my morning (little) cup of coffee pleases / delights me', *I liked his constructive comments* or *his constructive comments pleased me*. Though there does not exist a mental process verb of the *please* type for every verb of the *like* type, this bidirectionality is a general characteristic of mental processes, which has no parallel in material process clauses. (See Halliday, 1985/1994: 112–114, 116–117.)

self cannot be understood as a *distinct external* cause, i.e. as a typical external Agent (cf. *i zesti me pirazi* 'the heat's bothering me').[14]

Further evidence that such clauses are not clearly material processes comes from two closely related observations. To begin with, they cannot be probed by such questions as *ti su kani to xeri su*? 'what is your arm doing to you?'. Besides, despite their transitive structure and the presence of a Subject functioning as Agent, they cannot passivise either in Greek **ime ponemenos apo to xeri mu*, or in English, e.g. **I'm (being) hurt by my arm*, the personal pronoun having "more of a circumstantial function, somewhat like 'at me' or 'on me'" (see Halliday, 1998: 20). In Greek, it is not only that the particular process type (with any verb) cannot passivise (e.g. *to poδi mu me kei*, 'my leg is burning me' and **keyome apo to poδi mu* *'I'm being burnt by my leg') but, in addition, the verb *ponao* itself does not have a medio-passive morphology due to its syntactico-semantic properties.[15] In fact, the only form belonging to the medio-passive morphological paradigm is the participle *ponemenos* 'hurt', which occurs in ime 'be' + participle constructions, mostly as an adjectival form rather than a verbal one, e.g. *o omos mu ine poli ponemenos* 'my shoulder is very sore'.

Let us examine the following utterances. As we can see, in the second passage the patient originally communicates the sensation he experiences at the time of the medical consultation by means of the holistic *ponao*. It is only when the medical expert asks him about the nature of his pain that he refers to his knee as the Phenomenon / Agent in the painful sensation:

(29) P: endometaksi, *afto to poδi ke to γonato me ponai* liγaki.
meanwhile this the leg-NOM and the knee-NOM I-ACC hurt-PRS:3SG a-little
'Meanwhile, *this leg as well as the knee is hurting me* a little.'

14. This analysis of *to xeri mu me ponai* constructions has enabled me to interpret the intentionally funny effect produced by an expression that my late father used as a response to me when, as a child, I would complain that I was suffering from, say, a headache, by means of the construction *me ponai to kefali mu* 'my head is hurting me'. He would look at me very seriously and say '*pona to ki esi!*' '(you) hurt it too!', as if the Senser and Phenomenon roles could alternate and I could inflict pain on my head which could experience the sensation as a conscious being and I could in this way square up with my pain! Needless to say, the humour and affection expressed in my father's words definitely relieved my pain. After all, what he meant was that I could come face-to-face with my pain and master it, which was a very positive attitude.

15. According to Theophanopoulou-Kontou's analysis (1999), in the case of such unaccusative verbs as *anisixo* 'I worry', *sapizo* 'I rot / decay', *ljono* 'I melt', *kokinizo* 'I turn red', *mavrizo* 'I turn black', *arosteno* 'I fall ill', *peθeno* 'I die', etc., the absence of a medio-passive morphology is related to the semantics of the particular verbs which denote an internal process, and, therefore, exclude the presence of an external Agent. This analysis could also be extended to the verb *ponao* 'I hurt'.

(30) P: opos me piezete ponao. an m' afisete δen ponao.
as I-ACC squeeze-PRS:2PL hurt-PRS:1SG if I-ACC leave-PRS:2PL not hurt-PRS:1SG
'I'm hurting as you're squeezing me. If you stop squeezing me, I don't hurt.'
D: δen ponas? to iδio ke ja to alo poδi?
not hurt-PRS:2SG the same and for the other leg-ACC
'Aren't you hurting? Is it the same for the other leg, too?'
P: to iδjo ke eδo.
the same and here
'It's the same here, too.'
D: ke pos δilaδi, ti ponos?
and how that-is what pain-NOM
'And how, that is, what kind of pain?'
P: tora as pume liγo *me ponai to γonato mu.*
now let-IMP:IMPERS say-PFV:NON-PST:1PL a-bit I-ACC hurt-PRS:3SG the knee-NOM my
'Now let's say *my knee's hurting me* a bit.'

(31) ***me ponas / se ponao*?** No 8 of the paradigm
I-ACC hurt-PRS:2SG / you-ACC hurt-PRS:1SG
'you're hurting me' / 'am I hurting you?'

This is a typical material: effective process, i.e. one in which the 'doing', here the process of hurting, is extended to someone else and, hence, it is a process typically understood as focused in time. It is, therefore, transitive, on the one hand, and non-middle, on the other. Consequently, the participants involved are Goal and Actor, in transitive terms, and Medium and Agent, in ergative terms, represented by the suffering person and some other person, respectively. What is particular about such clauses is that normally the Agent / Actor is *unintentionally* 'doing' something, usually unpleasant, to the Medium / Goal. Evidence that these processes are material: effective comes from the possibility of using the probe *ti su kano tora, se ponao*? 'what am I doing to you now, am I hurting you?'

In the corpus of this study, they were very marginally observed, mainly in the course of a potentially pain-inducing examination or treatment where either the patient informed the medical expert that the latter was causing pain to him, or conversely, the doctor asked whether he was causing pain to the patient.

(32) D: se taleporo tora e?
you-ACC tire-PRS:1SG now eh
'Am I causing you any discomfort now, eh?'

P: aaaa!
ouch
'Ouch!'

D: eδo?
here
'Here?'

P: ne!
yes
'Yes!'

D: ke eδo ponas. a, ine lojika ta praγmata.
and here hurt-PRS:2SG ah be-PRS:3PL reasonable the things-NOM
'You're also hurting here. Ah, the situation is reasonable.'

P: mmm!
mmm
'Mmm!'

D: mmm!
mmm
'Mmm!'

P: mmm! ax *me poneses*, jatre mu, *me poneses*, trifto trifto liγo eki.
mmm ah I-ACC hurt-PST:2SG doctor-VOC my I-ACC hurt-PST:2SG rub-it-IMP:2SG rub-it-IMP:2SG a-bit there
'Mmm! Ah, *you hurt me*, (my) doctor, *you hurt me*, rub it, rub it a bit there.'

Though clauses having this structure passivise quite freely with other Greek verbs, with the verb *ponao* they cannot be converted into the passive, due to the absence of a medio-passive morphology of this verb discussed above (cf. *me piezis* 'you're pressurising me', *piezome apo sena* 'I'm being pressurised by you', *me esprokse enas aγnostos* 'a stranger pushed me', *sproxtika apo enan aγnosto* 'I was pushed by a stranger'). In that respect, such Greek constructions differ from the corresponding English ones, which can be turned into passive, e.g. *she got hurt by her dentist*.

(33) ***xtipisa to xeri mu*** No 9 of the paradigm
hit-PST:1SG the arm-ACC my
'I've hurt my arm'
[*not extracted from the data*]

Neither the pattern *xtipisa to xeri mu*, nor the next one *xtipisa* (*sto xeri mu*) (Nos 9 and 10 of the paradigm, which correspond more closely to the English expressions *I've hurt my arm* and *I've hurt myself* (*on the arm*), respectively) occurred at all in the corpus. It is noteworthy that, unlike all the other Greek constructions analysed here, neither of them contains a form of the verb *ponao*: the form *xtipisa* is the past tense of the verb *xtipo*, literally 'to hit'.

The unnaturalness of *ponesa*, the past tense of the verb *ponao*, rather than *xtipisa* 'I('ve) hit' in *xtipisa to xeri mu* 'I've hit my arm' must be sought in the semantic peculiarity of this two-participant construction, namely that it configures pain as a process unintentionally brought about by the person, i.e. the sufferer, to his own body part. The point at issue is that a body part, e.g. *to xeri mu*, could not be understood as a Senser, i.e. as an entity 'endowed with consciousness', one capable of 'sensing', and therefore it could not participate with this function in a mental: impacting process, with the sufferer as Phenomenon / Agent. Hence, the verb *ponesa* is unnatural in this Greek pattern. (See my note 14 above on *pona to ki esi!* '(you) hurt it too!'.) On the other hand, with the verb form *xtipisa* 'I('ve) hit' the process is interpreted as a material one with the sufferer as Actor and his body part as Goal, which makes *xtipisa to xeri mu* approximate most to the English *I've hurt my arm.*

It would be interesting to contrast the construction *xtipisa* / **ponesa to xeri mu* with its 'reverse' *to xeri mu me ponai* 'my arm's hurting me' (No 7 of the paradigm) discussed above, a mental: impacting process, involving the same two entities as participants in the process, i.e. the person suffering and his body part. What makes the Greek pattern *to xeri mu me ponai* and the corresponding English one *my arm's hurting me* perfectly grammatical is that the Senser is mapped onto the sufferer rather than the body part, which functions as the Phenomenon.

Though *xtipisa to xeri mu* can occur in the passive, like the English *I've hurt my arm*, it will also necessarily delete the Actor as Agent. Compare, *to xeri mu xtipiθike* (**apo mena*) and *my arm has been hurt* (**by me*). As Halliday (1998: 20) remarks, the ungrammaticality caused by the presence of an Agent-phrase reflects the fact that such constructions are "closely agnate to the next," (No 10 of the paradigm) in the sense that they are essentially reflexive in meaning (see below). The ungrammaticality of **to xeri mu xtipiθike apo mena* and of the corresponding English **my arm's been hurt by me* can be related to the impossibility of passivising the Greek *to xeri mu me ponai*, e.g. **ime ponemenos apo to xeri mu*, as well as the corresponding English *my arm is hurting me* (**I'm being hurt by my arm*). In both cases of ungrammatical passives it is primarily the presence of an Agent-phrase that accounts for their ungrammaticality, since, when omitted, the passive clauses become acceptable. It seems as if, by turning the person – in the first case – and the body part – in the second one – into Agent-phrases, the division / splitting of the sufferer into a body part 'at a distance from' his own self becomes even more dramatic and unnatural.

(34) ***xtipisa (sto xeri mu)*** No 10 of the paradigm
hit-PST:1SG (in-the arm-ACC my)
'I've hurt myself (on the arm)'
[*not extracted from the data*]

There was not a single instance of this construction in our data. Unlike the English configuration, where the presence of a second participant realised as the reflexive pronoun 'myself' clearly marks the process as material: effective / reflexive, there is no such marking in the Greek one, where the verb form, despite its active morphology, is understood as middle: reflexive, i.e. non-effective in voice. Once more, like the previous pattern (No 10 of the paradigm), this construction does not include a form of the verb *ponao*, which would rule out a reflexive interpretation. Like the corresponding English expression *I've hurt myself* (*on the arm*), the Greek pattern *xtipisa* (*sto xeri mu*) cannot passivise, due to its reflexive meaning. In both languages the body part, in the form of a prepositional phrase, is not construed as a nuclear participant, but rather as a circumstance of Location. It is this configuration of the body part as a less central component of the process that excludes from this construction the direct 'confrontation' between the sufferer and some body part in roles of equal status that seem to bring them vis-à-vis as separate entities.

(35) ***afto ponai*** No 11 of the paradigm
that-NOM hurt-PRS:3SG
'that hurts'

I suggest that the presence of only one participant in *afto ponai* 'that hurts' makes it plausible to interpret this Greek construction primarily as a mental process, one in which only the Phenomenon as the source of pain, i.e. *afto*, is present in the clause, while the Senser is simply implied (cf. *afto enoxli* 'that annoys'). My proposed interpretation of this configuration is motivated by the understanding of mental processes as a category which always potentially involves both a Senser and a Phenomenon but need not necessarily include both in the clause, i.e. any of the two may be only implicitly present (see Halliday, 1985/1994: 118). Thus, I propose that *afto*, which could be a particular movement, an activity, an instrument or a treatment, is understood as Phenomenon in a mental process where the Medium / Senser, i.e. the sufferer, may remain unspecified. This understanding of *afto ponai*, I suggest, gains further support from Halliday's (1998: 21) interpretation of the corresponding English expression *that hurts* as less focused in time, which is typical of mental processes, despite the fact that he does not analyse the particular pattern as a mental process. Consider:

(36) D: iparxi, exete vri *kati* etsi, *pu ponai* poli ektos ap' to skipsimo?
there-is, have PRS:2PL find-PFV something-ACC like-this which hurt-PRS:3SG a-lot besides the bending-NOM
'Is there, have you found out *anything else* besides bending *that hurts* a lot?'

(37) P: *ke i δio akrees θesis ponane* poli.
and the two extreme-NOM positions-NOM hurt-PRS:3PL a-lot
'*Both extreme positions hurt* a lot.'

Alternatively, in the light of Halliday's interpretation of the English pattern, the Greek construction *afto ponai* could be construed as relational: attributive, one in which pain is understood as a quality, an Attribute, in conflation with the Process, like construction *to xeri mu ponai* 'my arm hurts' (i.e. No 1 of the paradigm). The important difference between *to xeri mu ponai* and *afto ponai* is that in the latter the syntactic Subject of *ponai*, i.e. *afto* 'that', is not a body part functioning as the Carrier of the Attribute but, rather, it is another, inanimate, entity such as an object or process, construed as the Agent. What makes the construction *afto ponai* quite special according to this analysis is that, despite the presence of an agency feature in the form of the structural function Agent – which is typical of effective (i.e. non-middle) two-participant clauses – there is no linguistically realised second participant here. Thus, this is neither a typical relational attributive clause nor a typical agentive one, but it shares features of both. Hence, the Attribute which is conflated with the Process is understood as the ability to cause pain. In other words, *afto* 'that' is ascribed the quality of being painful, in the sense of being capable of inducing pain, the entity to which the pain is extended not actually being at issue (cf. *afto leroni* 'that dirties', *afti i alifi δen lekiazi* 'this ointment does not stain').[16] E.g.:

(38) D: δen θelume na kanete enesis. *ponane ki aftes.*
not want-PRS:1PL to-PARTCL do-PRS:2PL injections-ACC hurt- PRS:3PL and these-NOM
'We don't want you to have injections. *They also hurt.*'

(39) ***afto me ponai*** Nos 12 & 12a of the paradigm
that-NOM I-ACC hurt-PRS:3SG
'that's hurting me'

This is one of the two constructions observed in the Greek corpus that do not correspond to any of the pain expressions of Halliday's paradigm. Compared to *afto ponai*, it differs with respect to the presence of *me* 'me' as a second participant.

16. Theophanopoulou-Kontou (personal communication) suggested that these are unergative structures, i.e. having an external argument only, due to the omission of the direct object, according to Levin and Rappaport Hovav's (1995) analysis.

Moreover, wherever this structure occurs in the data it refers to processes with clear beginnings and endings, as is typical of material processes. I suggest, therefore, that it could be construed as a material: effective process, with the person as Goal and the other entity – an object or process – as Agent / Actor. Hence, in this pain construal the sufferer is seen as experiencing pain caused at a particular time by an external inanimate entity, such as a medical instrument or a pain-inducing activity (cf. *afto me tsimbai* 'that's pricking me', *afto me yaryαlai* 'that's tickling me').

(40) P: ine ekino to simio pu pono para poli. para poli.
be-PRS:3SG that the point-NOM where hurt-PRS:1SG very much very much
'It's that point where I hurt a lot. A lot.'
D: *se ponai afto pu su kano?*
you-ACC hurt-PRS:3SG that which you-GEN do-PRS:1SG
'*Is what I'm doing to you hurting you?*'
P: e?
eh
'Eh?'
D: *se ponai afto pu su kano?*
you-ACC hurt-PRS:3SG that which you-GEN do-PRS:1SG
'*Is what I'm doing to you hurting you?*'

(41) D: ja kane mu pros ta piso. xalarotiko? ja kane mu opos ise strofi pros tin ali plevra.
just do-IMP:2SG I-GEN towards the back relaxing just do-IMP:2SG I-GEN as be-PRS:2SG turn-ACC towards the other side-ACC
'Just move backwards for me. Relaxing? Do me a favour and turn to the other side, as you are.'
P: ne, e, afto δiskolo.
yes eh this difficult-NOM
'Yes, eh, this (is) difficult.'
D: mmm… *i plaja kampsi ke δeksia strofi se ponai…*
mmm the side bending-NOM and right turn-NOM you-ACC hurt-PRS:3SG
'Mmm… *bending sideways and turning towards the right is what's hurting you…*'
P: *me ponai*, ne.
I-ACC hurt-PRS:3SG yes
'*It's hurting me*, yes.'

The two dialogues above contain instances of this pattern. In the first one, the health care professional repeatedly employs it in the course of an activity (a movement, perhaps) to find out whether it causes pain to the patient. In the second case, the medical expert uses it to name the particular pain-inducing movement, while the patient's response actually echoes the structure.

(42) ***me ponai (eδo)*** Nos 13 & 14 of the paradigm
I-ACC hurt-PRS:3SG:IMPERS (here)
'it hurts / it's hurting me (here)'

This is the second Greek construction not corresponding to any English pattern featuring in Halliday's account. Here pain is construed as a mental process, either typically unbounded in time (No 13, mental: effective), or more focused in time (No 14, mental: impacting), which is less typical of such processes. In both cases, the third-person singular impersonal verb suffix functions as impersonal Phenomenon in the same way that *it* is configured in the English translation equivalents 'it hurts me' and 'it's hurting me'. Just as *they* cannot replace *it* in English, the plural *ponane* is not a possible variant (**me ponane* *'they hurt / are hurting me'). The other participant of the process, the person *me* 'me', is the typical one in a mental clause, i.e. the Senser (cf. *me tsuzi* (*eδo*) 'it stings me (here)', *me troi* (*eδo*), 'it itches me (here')).

In the dialogues below, we observe two instances of the impersonal *me ponai* pattern. Once more, in the first extract, the patient initially expresses his pain holistically by means of the form *ponao*. In the second one, he first names the existence of his pain in terms of the impersonal existential *ponai*, he then continues with the equally impersonal mental: impacting *me ponai*, and, finally, he is able to communicate his sensation more explicitly and makes use of the material: effective construction *tora me ponai i piesi pu mu askis* 'now it's the pressure you're exercising on me that's hurting me.'

(43) P: tora ponao.
now hurt-PRS:1SG
'I'm hurting now.'
D: pu?
where
'Where?'
P: *me ponai* ston karpo.
I-ACC hurt-PRS:3SG:IMPERS in-the wrist-ACC
'*It's hurting me* in the wrist.'
D: eδo mesa? eδo?
here inside here
'Inside here? Here?'

P: ne, eδo.
yes here
'Yes, here.'

D: ke apo 'δo pano ponai δilaδi?
and from here above hurt-PRS:3SG:IMPERS that-is
'Do you mean it's hurting up here as well?'

(44) P: ne, ponai.
yes hurt-PRS:3SG:IMPERS
'Yes, it's hurting.'

D: ponai eki.
hurt-PRS:3SG:IMPERS there
'It's hurting there.'

P: liγo *me ponai*. tora me ponai i piesi pu mu askis.
a-bit I-ACC hurt-PRS:3SG:IMPERS now I-ACC hurt-PRS:3SG the pressure-NOM that I-GEN exercise-PRS:2SG
'*It's hurting me* a bit. Now it's the pressure you're exercising on me that's hurting me.'

If we relate the impersonal mental process *me ponai* with the other impersonal construction in the data, namely the existential (existing or occurring) *ponai*, we observe that it is the presence of *me* in the former that marks the difference between these two pain configurations. To be more precise, the absence of a second participant in the existential *ponai* does not allow the third-person singular suffix incorporated in the verb form to function as anything else but an impersonal Setting. On the other hand, the existence of *me* in the mental *me ponai* brings the sufferer as Senser onto the scene, making it possible to construe the impersonal element as a more vital participant than the Setting, namely, as the Phenomenon, i.e. 'what is sensed'. Being impersonal, however, 'what is sensed' cannot acquire the status of Agent like *afto* in the case of *afto ponai* 'that hurts' and *afto me ponai* 'that's hurting me'.

6.4.1 Concluding remarks

Our data analysis has revealed that pain as process in Greek enters into figures of almost every type, namely, 'doing and happening', 'sensing' or 'being'. Moreover, in its processual framing, pain is mostly understood as dwelling in the sufferer's self configured holistically (56.66% of all collected verbal patterns), since in only about one fifth of the data (20.78%) is a part of the sufferer's body represented as the locus of pain, while in one more fifth of the material (19.66%) pain appears as residing in an abstract, impersonal, non-specific, virtual Setting.

Thus, the functional account of the Greek data has provided empirical evidence bearing out the argument expressed by Wittgenstein (1953/1989: 98, § 286) that it is absurd to assume that it is the body rather than the sufferer that 'feels' pain:

> But isn't it absurd to say of a *body* that it has pain? – And why does one feel an absurdity in that? In what sense is it true that my hand does not feel pain, but I in my hand?
> What sort of issue is: Is it the *body* that feels pain? – How is it to be decided? What makes it plausible to say that it is *not* the body? – Well, something like this: if someone has a pain in his hand, then the hand does not say so (unless it writes it) and one does not comfort the hand, but the sufferer: one looks into his face.

From his functional linguistic perspective, but very much along the same line of reasoning, Halliday (1998: 27) also argues that:

> The one who suffers pain is always a conscious being, even if the entity in which the pain is actualized is merely a part of the sufferer's body. Pain is ascribed precisely to the category of beings that are referred to pronominally as *he/she*, not as *it*.

To conclude, from the analysis of the diverse processual configurations of pain drawn from our Greek doctor-patient dialogues it emerges that, overall, these have a stronger expressive rather than descriptive function. What is more, I propose that intransitive first-person *ponao* 'I hurt' / 'I'm hurting' and impersonal third-person *ponai* 'it hurts' / 'it's hurting' pain utterances often function in the same way as pain exclamations, with which they are actually observed to co-occur or alternate in the data. Drawing on Foolen's (1997) study of the expressive function of language and his proposed analysis of the communication of emotional content, I suggest that these pain utterances could be identified with a potential direct linguistic expression of pain. Hence, such instances of the specific verb forms could be schematically represented by assuming positions next to interjections, which are the linguistic signs positioned most closely to the expressive pole of the proposed continuum – comprising automatic non-linguistic pain reactions, e.g. cries / groans / screams – while the remaining patterns could be symbolically arranged in intermediate positions along the expressive-descriptive axis of the scale. To illustrate the gradience that I assume the expressive function of the processual framing of pain to have, I propose the following symbolic arrangement of the collected patterns as we move from the expressive to the descriptive pole: *ponao* (*eδo*) 'I hurt / I'm hurting (here)' > *ponai* (*eδo*) 'it hurts / it's hurting (here)' > *me ponai* (*eδo*) 'it hurts me / it's hurting me (here)' > *to xeri mu* (*mu*) *ponai* 'my arm hurts / my arm's hurting (in me)' > *to xeri mu me ponai* 'my arm's hurting me' > *afto ponai* 'that hurts' > (*afto*) *me ponai* 'that's hurting me' > *me ponas* / *se ponao*? 'you're hurting me' / 'am I hurting you?'.

CHAPTER 7

The construal of pain as thing-participant

7.1 Introduction

In what follows we shall be concerned with the construal of pain as thing, linguistically realised in Greek by *ponos* nominal expressions, and the relevant constructions observed in the corpus. We shall first examine the lexico-grammatical properties of *ponos* and the syntactic configurations it appears in, in the light of Halliday's (1985/94) functional approach, assuming applicability of his paradigm to Greek, at least to a large extent (see Lascaratou and Marmaridou, 2005).

Adopting Halliday's functional analysis of pain, we are indirectly initiated into the metaphorical understanding of this experiential domain of everyday life, as there are two important aspects of his account pointing to this direction. On the one hand, Halliday (1998: 11) himself establishes his object of investigation in metaphorical terms when he considers pain, which is an experience, i.e. an event, to be a thing, an entity, or a participant in a process. On the other, confronted with the complexities of pain as an area of human experience, he intuitively describes it not simply as being "unpleasant" and "distressing", but as having the characteristics of a lurking, threatening, enemy that is "arbitrary and ruthless" to the sufferer, and ultimately "potentially life-destroying" (*ibid.*: 29). However, what becomes crucial in our study of *ponos* is that, despite the metaphorical structuring of Halliday's intuitions, his analysis proper does not actually provide any lexico-grammatical evidence for their expression.[1]

The thorough examination of the doctor-patient dialogues on which the analysis presented in Chapter 8 is based will provide further evidence in support of the claim originally put forward in Lascaratou and Marmaridou (2005) that "Halliday's insights are justified when we investigate the conceptual basis of pain language, thereby grounding the functional paradigm in a cognitive semantics approach." Thus, after I have completed a detailed structural and functional account of *ponos* nominal constructions in this chapter, I shall examine the metaphorical representation of pain in such constructions in the next chapter. The refinement of the analysis

1. As we shall see below in our discussion of the central role of metaphor in pain language (Chapter 8), these intuitions are borne out by medical and social scientists' accounts.

of the conceptual structure of pain language that I will propose will be grounded on an enhancement of the theoretical framework, by means of e.g. a revised application of Talmy's (1988) force dynamic schema, Kövecses's (2000 and forth.) analysis of the conceptual structure of emotion and pain, as well as the concept of 'embodiment'. Hence, on the basis of a more elaborate analysis of the Greek pain data, I will be able to argue that specific-level pain metaphors are instantiations of such a general metaphor as PAIN IS A FORCE which parallels the overarching generic-level master metaphor EMOTIONS ARE FORCES; I will also argue that specific-level pain metaphors are constrained by the universal aspects of the human body's functioning in pain, i.e. by the particular types of actual or potential tissue damage and their accompanying sensory effects.

Finally, my analysis of the lexico-grammatical properties of *ponos* and the interpretation of the related nominal constructions from both a functional and a cognitive semantic perspective will highlight the descriptive, reportive and objectifying character of such structures.

7.2 Grammatically construed semantic properties of *ponos*

Let us now proceed to see how *ponos* is construed in lexico-grammatical terms using relevant data from the doctor-patient dialogues. My analysis will be framed on the basis of what Halliday (1998: 11–13) identifies as seven 'grammatical properties' or 'semantic features' associated with pain as thing. In fact, Halliday uses both terms interchangeably to refer to what can be understood as grammatically construed semantic properties of pain, namely, that pain

a. may be construed as a bounded or an unbounded thing
b. is a possession which may be acquired, received, owned, and lost
c. has temporal location and extent
d. has accompanying conditions, grammatically construed as a temporal nexus
e. has variable location within the body
f. varies in intensity, and
g. manifests variable qualities.

7.2.1 *Ponos* as a bounded or an unbounded thing

As in English, pain in Greek may be construed both as a bounded or an unbounded thing, i.e. it appears both as a countable and a mass noun, though in Greek its construal as a bounded entity seems to prevail over its understanding as an unbounded one.[2] When it behaves as a bounded entity, *ponos* may be accompanied by a determiner, e.g. the definite or indefinite article, i.e. *o* / *ton* 'the'-NOM/-ACC or *enas* / *enan* 'a'-NOM/-ACC, e.g. (1) and (2), a demonstrative, e.g. *aftos* / *afton* 'this'-NOM/-ACC as in (3), a possessive form, e.g. *o δikos mu* 'my own' or *mu* 'my' as in (4), it may pluralise, e.g. (5), or it may have a diminutive suffix attached to it, e.g. *pon-akus* or *pon-akia* as in (6).[3] On the other hand, the unbounded understanding of *ponos* is expressed in its bare singular form, e.g. (7)-(9). As Halliday (*ibid.*: 11) points out, pain shifts from one category to the other, its complex nature being the main factor underlying its double construal. In Greek this shifting is equally observed in *ponos* compound forms, such as *ponokefalos* 'headache', *kiloponos* 'tummy pain', *ponoδondos* 'toothache', *nevroponos* 'pain in a nerve'. Finally, this understanding of *ponos* as either a bounded or an unbounded entity will be shown to have a central role in the interpretation of constructions where it is configured as the syntactic object of the verbs *exo* 'have', *esθanome* 'feel', and *njoθo* 'feel' (see section 8.2.1).

In (1)-(6) *ponos* is represented as a bounded thing:

(1) P: otan exo *ton ponokefalo*, δen pino.
when have-PRS:1SG the headache-ACC not drink-PRS:1SG
'When I have *the headache*, I don't drink.'

(2) P: itan *enas* aljotikos *ponos*.
be-PST:3SG a different pain-NOM
'That was *a* different *pain*.'

(3) P: mi mu ksanamilisis ja *afton ton pono*!
not I-GEN talk-again-PFV:NON-PST:2SG for this the pain-ACC
'Don't talk to me about *this pain* again!'

(4) D: pite mu lipon, irθate ja *ton pono sas*?
tell-IMP:2PL I-GEN then come-PST:2PL for the pain-ACC your
'Tell me then, have you come here for *your pain*?'

2. Langacker (1987: 203) contends that the count / mass distinction is notionally based: a count noun "designates a region that is specifically construed as being bounded within the scope of predication in a primary domain" whereas a mass noun "designates a region that is not so construed."

3. From my preliminary on-going exploration of *ponos* constructions in the present version of the Corpus of Greek Texts (CGT) – an extensive (7,280,086 words / tokens), non-specialised, representative corpus of (spoken and written) Greek which is still in the process of being compiled – it appears that the majority of the collected plural forms of the noun *ponos* (92.50%) denote physical rather than mental pain. I suggest that the pluralisation of *ponos* denoting physical pain and, hence, its assumed boundedness / countability indicates that physical pain is perceived as a concrete rather than an abstract entity.

(5) P: oxi, δen ixa *ponus* kaθolu.
no not have-PST:1SG pains-ACC at-all
'No, I didn't have *any pains* at all.'

(6) P: exo *ponakia*, opos sas eksijisa.
have-PRS:1SG little-pains-ACC as you-GEN:PL explain-PST:1SG
'I have *little pains*, as I explained to you.'

Utterances (7)-(9) are examples of *ponos* as an unbounded thing:

(7) P: δen boro na po *pono* afto to praγma.
not can-PRS:1SG to-PARTCL call-PFV:NON-PST:1SG this the thing-ACC
'I can't call this thing *pain*.'

(8) D: exete *ponokefalo*?
have-PRS:2PL headache-ACC
'Do you have *a headache*?'

(9) D: njoθis eki *pono*?
feel-PRS:2SG there pain-ACC
'Do you feel *pain* there?'

7.2.2 *Ponos* as a possession: Acquired, received, owned, and lost

Pain is a possession which may be acquired (10), received (11), owned (12)-(13), and lost (15).[4] However, unlike the case of typical possessions where the possessor strives to acquire something and then to preserve it, here the sufferer acquires, or is given, an undesired possession which he struggles hard to free himself from, being unable to "give it away, or put it back wherever it came from" (Halliday, *ibid.*: 4). Even more tragically, as our data illustrate, if the 'owner' manages to get rid of his pain, he never knows when he may 'reacquire' it, in which case he immediately recognises it as a possession that has become familiar to him, e.g. (14). The use of possessive markers, mainly used in our material by doctors when requesting information about the patient's condition, contributes to the understanding of pain as a possession, for example (16) and (17). Surprisingly, however, such possessive modifiers of *ponos* were found to be overall quite marginally used.

(10) P: *arxisa na exo* frixtus ponus.
start-PST:1SG to-PARTCL have-PRS:1SG terrible-ACC pains-ACC
'*I started having* terrible pains.'

4. The conceptualisation of pain as a possession (e.g. *have (a) pain, give pain to someone*) is also proposed by Peters (2004: 199) in his historical semantic account of English pain words.

(11) P: δen ksero ti mu *prokali* tus ponus.
not know-PRS:1SG what-NOM I-GEN cause-PRS:3SG the pains:ACC
'I don't know what *causes* the pains to me.'

(12) D: ke ektos, ipame, apo ton pono stin mesi, *exete* ke ton pono stin kilia.
and apart say-PST:1PL from the pain-ACC in-the low-back-ACC have-PRS:2PL and the pain-ACC in-the tummy-ACC
'And, as we said, apart from the low back pain, you also *have* the pain in the tummy.'

(13) P: exune fiji ta spirakia ke *exi mini* o ponos.
have-PRS:3PL go-PFV the little-spots:NOM and have-PRS:3SG remain-PFV the pain-NOM
'The little spots have gone and the pain *has remained*.'

(14) P: jati aftus tus ponus tus *ksanaixa* ke perpatusa δiplomeni sta δio.
because these the pains:ACC they-ACC have-again-IPFV:1SG and walk-IPFV:1SG bent-NOM in-the-ACC:PL two
'Because *I've had* these pains *again* and I could only walk bent in two.'

(15) P: prin to xirurjio *ixa* mesopona, ma *eperasan*…
before the surgery-ACC have-IPFV:1SG lumbar-pains:ACC but pass-PST:3PL
'Before the surgery, I *had* lumbar pains, but they *have passed*…'

(16) D: emaθes na zis me *ton pono su*, afton ton liγo pono…
learn-PST:2SG to-PARTCL live-PRS:2SG with the pain-ACC your this the little pain-ACC
'You have learnt to live with *your pain*, this little pain…'

(17) P: o ponos ezvise, o alos, *o δikos mu*.
the pain-NOM fade-away-PST:3SG the other-NOM the mine my
'The pain has faded away, the other, *my own*.'

We will be considering the possessive construal of pain in more detail both in section 7.3 below, where a functional account of the various types of figure where *ponos* enters as a participant will be presented, and in the next chapter, where a thorough analysis of the semantic features of *exo* + *ponos* constructions will provide the necessary basis for a cognitive semantic account of the metaphorical understanding of *ponos* as an alienable possession and, ultimately, its conceptualisation as an objectified entity.

7.2.3 The temporal location and extent of *ponos*

Pain may be specified in terms of temporal location, e.g. (18) and extent, e.g. (19). In fact, medical experts typically request information about the temporal characteristics of the patient's pain as these may contribute to the understanding of its nature and origin. It emerges from the corpus dialogues that health care professionals attribute great importance to the particular time of the day (or night) when pain occurs or becomes worse, thus, assuming that pain may appear as a series of events taking place in a regularly repeated order, i.e. it recurs in cycles as in examples (20) and (21). As Halliday (1998: 12) notes for English, the duration of pain may also be metaphorically expressed as a quality in the form of an adjective (e.g. *sinexomenos* / *sinexis* 'continuous', *δiarkis* 'constant', *monimos* 'permanent', *xronios* 'chronic') having the function of Epithet or Attribute (see examples (22)-(23), and (24)-(25), respectively).[5]

(18) D: isaste kala *mexri ton iulio*? δen ixate aftus tus ponus?
be-PST:2PL well until the July-ACC not have-IPFV:2PL these the pains:ACC
'Were you well *until July*? Didn't you have these pains?'

(19) D: ke *poso kratuse* aftos o ponos?
and how long last-IPFV:3SG this the pain-NOM
'And *how long* did this pain last?'
P: poles fores *ke δekapende* ixe kratisi.
many times-ACC and fifteen have-PST:3SG last-PFV
'Quite often it had lasted *as long as fifteen days*.'

(20) D: *to vraδi* o ponos xiroterevi i *to proi* ine xiroteros? *pote* nomizete, i δen exi…?
the evening-ACC the pain-NOM become-worse-PRS:3SG or the morning-ACC be-PRS:3SG worse-NOM when think-PRS:2PL or not have-PRS:3SG
'Does the pain become worse *in the evening* or is it worse *in the morning*? *When* do you think, or doesn't it have…?'

5. A clarification of the terms Epithet and Classifier (see below) would be useful here. Thus, according to Halliday (1985/1994: 184–185), the Epithet "indicates some quality of the subset, e.g. *old, long, blue, fast*" while the Classifier "indicates a particular subclass of the thing in question, e.g. *electric trains, passenger trains, wooden trains, toy trains*." The line between Epithet and Classifier, he remarks, is not very sharply drawn (though there are important differences), as there are cases where the same word may have either of the two functions, with a different semantic effect: e.g. in *fast trains* the word *fast* is either Epithet, i.e. trains that go fast, or Classifier, i.e. trains classified as expresses.

P: ðen exi *orario*, ðen exi *orario*, oxi.
not have-PRS:3SG schedule-ACC not have-PRS:3SG schedule-ACC no
'It has no *schedule*, it has no *schedule*, no.'

(21) P: eðo me ponese poli…
here I-ACC hurt-PST:3SG:IMPERS a-lot
'It hurt me a lot here…'

D: *sinexos*?
continuously
'*Continuously*?'

P: enas *sinexomenos* ponos.
a continuous pain-NOM
'A *continuous* pain.'

D: exi eksarsis i etsi ine *sinexja sinexja* to iðio?
have-PRS:3SG peaks-ACC or like-this be-PRS:3SG continuously continuously the same-NOM
'Does it have peaks or is it the same *all the time*?'

P: tora exo *ke tris meres* pu me exi peθani ston pono. poli pono.
now have-PRS:1SG and three days-ACC that I-ACC have-PRS:3SG:IMPERS die-PFV in-the pain-ACC much pain-ACC
'I've been dying from pain *for at least three days* now. A lot of pain.'

(22) P: ðen ine *ðiarkis* ponos…
not be-PRS:3SG constant pain-NOM
'It is not a *constant* pain…'

(23) P: …afto pja exi jini enas ponos toso *monimos* jati ton exo *pende xronia sinexja*.
this-NOM by-now have-PRS:3SG become-PFV a pain-NOM so permanent-NOM because it-ACC have-PRS:1SG five years-ACC continuously
'…by now, this has become such a *permanent* pain because I've had it *for five years incessantly*.'

(24) P: …pleon aftos o ponos exi jini *xronios*.
by-now this the pain-NOM have-PRS:3SG become-PFV chronic-NOM
'…by now, this pain has become *chronic*.'

(25) D: ine *sinexis* aftos o ponos?
be-PRS:3SG continuous-NOM this the pain-NOM
'Is this pain *continuous*?'

7.2.4 The accompanying conditions of *ponos*: A temporal nexus

As the extracts (26) and (27) from our dialogues illustrate, in addition to being specified in the form of adverbials or adjectives, the temporal properties of the pain experience may additionally be identified in terms of accompanying conditions, grammatically construed as a temporal nexus. Interestingly, the situation described in the Greek doctor-patient conversation under (27) is quite similar to the one specified in the English medical consultation dialogue provided by Halliday (1998: 13): in both, the patient complains about suffering when he stands up / is standing up. In the Greek example the patient is very eager to describe his suffering conditions and lists them all explicitly in the form of a multiple temporal nexus.

(26) P: *an viasto ke trekso liyo*, esθanome ton pono pali.
if hurry-up-PFV:NON-PST:1SG and run-PFV:NON-PST:1SG a-little feel-PRS:1SG the pain-ACC again
'*If I am in a hurry and rush*, I feel the pain again.'

(27) D: pos njoθis *to proi otan sikonese*?
how feel-PRS:2SG the morning-ACC when get-up-PRS:2SG
'How do you feel *in the morning when you get up*?'

P: *to proi* δen esθanome pono.
the morning-ACC not feel-PRS:1SG pain-ACC
'*In the morning* I don't feel pain.'

D: *pote*? o ponos su *pote* arxizi?
when the pain-NOM your when start-PRS:3SG
'*When*? *When* does your pain start?'

P: o ponos arxizi *otan sikoθo*…
the pain-NOM start-PRS:3SG when stand-up-PFV:NON-PST:1SG
'The pain starts *when I stand up*…'

D: ne.
yes
'Yes.'

P: *ke kaθiso orθia*, p.x. *an skipso ja na kano kati, an prospaθiso na metakiniso kati*. p.x. *na paro tin karekla ke na tin metakiniso sta pende metra*.
and stand-PFV:NON-PST:1SG upright e.g. if bend-PFV:NON-PST:1SG to do-PFV:NON-PST:1SG something if try-PFV:NON-PST:1SG to move-PFV:NON-PST:1SG something e.g. to get-PFV:NON-PST:1SG the chair-ACC and to it-ACC move-PFV:NON-PST:1SG in-the five metres-ACC
'*and straighten up my body*, e.g. *if I bend to do something, if I try to move something*, e.g. *to get the chair and move it as far as five metres*.'

7.2.5 The variable location of *ponos* within the body

When pain is linguistically realised through the noun *ponos*, its variable location within the body is very often specified either by means of adverbials, such as *eδo* / *eki* 'here' / 'there', or a locative of place, e.g. (28)-(32), whereby location is represented as a circumstance, or in the form of a compound noun specifying the painful body part, e.g. *ponokefalos* 'headache', *mesopona* 'low back pains'. In the corpus, two more formal, medical terms deriving from the archaic form *alyos* 'pain' also occurred, namely, *osfialjia* (*osfis* 'loins' + *alyos* 'pain') 'lumbar pain' and *isxialjia* (*isxion* 'hip' + *alyos* 'pain') 'sciatica', which are not, however, always familiar to patients, as the dialogue under (33) reveals. In addition to these main construals of the locus of pain, there is another option in English, namely, a construction such as *tummy pains* where the location appears as Classifier in a nominal group with *pain* as Thing (Halliday, 1998: 12).[6] Such sequences of two nouns where one functions as a modifier of the other not being productive in Greek, this additional construal of pain location does not occur. However, in Greek we also observe cases where it is the locative of place which functions as a modifier of the noun *ponos* (e.g. *o ponos mu* <u>*apo ton yofo*</u> 'my pain from the thigh', see also (29)). Furthermore, in our material there are a few instances of the adjective *topikos* 'local' and the pseudo-participle *endopizmenos* 'localised' grammatically representing the location of pain either as Epithet or Attribute, e.g. (30). Most importantly, we notice that in our data the location of pain is quite often not simply identified as a particular spot or part of the body but, rather, as an area extending from one point to another in the sufferer's body, as some kind of 'path' through which pain 'travels', e.g. (30)-(33). As we shall see in Chapter 8, this construal of the locus of pain is closely related to the understanding of *ponos* as a moving entity, which is the basic metaphorical configuration motivating a number of other metaphors whereby *ponos* is personified, taking on agent-like properties, and can, thus, be conceptualised as an external, volitional aggressor.

(28) D: o ponos ine mono *sto yonato*?
the pain-NOM be-PRS:3SG only in-the knee-ACC
'Is the pain only *in the knee*?'

(29) D: …ji' afto ke irθate se mas eδo, δilaδi ji' afton *ton pono eδo sti stomatiki kilotita*?
for-this and come-PST:2PL to we-ACC here that-is for this the pain-ACC here in-the oral cavity-ACC
'…is that actually why you've come to us here, that is, for this *pain here in the oral cavity*?'

6. See note 5 above.

(30) D: aftos eδo o ponos, ti ponos ine? ine *eδo topikos i pai ke mexri kato*?
this here the pain-NOM what pain-NOM be-PRS:3SG be-PRS:3SG here local or go-PRS:3SG and right-to down
'This pain here, what kind of pain is it? Is it *local, here*, or *does it also move right down*?'

(31) P: ksekinai *apo to zverko* ke kataliji *eδo, stus krotafus.*
start-PRS:3SG from the neck-ACC and extend-PRS:3SG here in-the temples-ACC
'It starts *from the neck* and extends up to *here, in the temples.*'

(32) P: exo pono *sti mesi…*
have-PRS:1SG pain-ACC in-the low-back-ACC
'I've got a *low back* pain…'

D: ne.
yes
'Yes.'

P: *…eδo xamila… mexri to poδi* mu pjani…
here low right-to the leg-ACC my extend-PRS:3SG
'*…here quite low…* it extends *right to my leg…*'

(33) D: *isxialjia* sas kani?
sciatica-ACC you-GEN:PL cause-PRS:3SG
'Does it cause you *sciatica*?'

P: e?
hm
'What?'

D: *isxialjia* sas kani?
sciatica-ACC you-GEN:PL cause-PRS:3SG
'Does it cause you *sciatica*?'

P: δen ksero.
not know-PRS:1SG
'I don't know.'

D: *pai kato* o ponos etsi *sto poδi*?
go-PRS:3SG down the pain-NOM like-this in-the leg-ACC
'Does the pain somehow *go down to the leg* like this?'

P: oso δen boro na perpatiso.
so-much not can-PRS:1SG to walk-PFV:NON PST:1SG
'So much that I can't walk.'

I shall close the examination of the grammatically construed semantic properties of *ponos*, with a discussion of its variable intensity and qualities, which are very significant and, quite often, interrelated aspects of the pain experience.

7.2.6 The degree of intensity and the variable qualities of *ponos:* Mapping the Greek data onto the McGill Pain Questionnaire (MPQ)

As my analysis of Greek pain descriptors will show, degree of intensity and quality of pain cannot always be easily distinguished from each other, but rather they seem to merge in the form of adjectives, which are metonymically derived metaphorical representations of the sensory aspect of pain, often combining semantic features related to both intensity and quality: e.g. *ylikos* 'sweet', which can be understood as having a particular quality and/or mild intensity, and *oksis* 'sharp', which inherently combines quality and severe intensity. (See relevant discussion below and in Chapter 8, section 8.2.3.) What is more, even in terms of quality, some pain descriptors can be interpreted as expressing more than one properties, e.g. *vaθis* 'deep', which refers to a spatial characteristic of the sensation but may also imply sharpness, by virtue of its ability to be sensed deep in the body. Moreover, given that, as was noted above, duration of pain may also be metaphorically configured as a quality realised through an adjective, e.g. *sinexis* 'continuous', *monimos* 'permanent', it is a further feature of pain that may merge with quality, e.g. in *xronios* 'chronic'. DeSouza and Frank (2000: 217) observe that, unlike what interviewers might expect, most subjects resist describing intensity of pain by means of a single concept and provide instead multifaceted accounts, which may be due to their inability to discriminate between various components of pain. Thus, for example, subjects may envisage the amount of pain they experience as a concept of time, while others may use spatial characteristics to quantify their pain. It seems plausible to assume that the degree of this indeterminacy of categories is, to some extent, dependent on language-specific factors.

It is the complexity of assessing the degree of intensity and the various qualities of the pain sensation that motivated Melzack and Torgerson's (1971) attempt to develop new approaches to the problem of describing and measuring pain, by devising lists of descriptive words that provided the basis for the subsequent development of the McGill Pain Questionnaire (MPQ) (Melzack, 1975), one of the most widely used multidimensional pain measures over the past thirty years. In its extended version, the MPQ comprises 78 descriptive adjectives categorised into three major classes and 20 subclasses. The classes are: a) words describing *sensory qualities* in terms of temporal, spatial, pressure, thermal, and other properties,[7] e.g. *beating, flashing, scalding*, and *stinging*, b) words describing *affective qualities*, i.e. negative emotional reactions, in terms of tension, fear, and autonomic properties, e.g. *suffocating, frightful*, and *vicious*, and c) *evaluative* words describing the subjective overall intensity of pain, e.g. *annoying, intense*, and *unbearable*.

Given that the MPQ proved to be time-consuming and, in certain cases, unnecessarily detailed, in 1987 Melzack constructed its short form (SFMPQ), whose main component consists of 15 adjectives, of which 11 describe sensory pain properties and 4 affective ones. Pain intensity is measured on a four-point rating scale (*none, mild, moderate*, and *severe*) by the patient himself who assigns the appropriate score to those descriptors that best represent his painful sensation. Hence, both qualitative and quantitative information is simultaneously collected. The questionnaire includes a further verbal and numerical rating scale, the Present Pain Index (PPI), a five-point scale (*mild, discomforting, distressing, horrible*, and *excruciating*) used for the description of pain intensity while completing the questionnaire.

In its short form, the MPQ has recently been translated into Greek (GR-SFMPQ, see Georgoudis, Watson and Oldham, 2000 and Georgoudis, Oldham and Watson, 2001). To make our discussion of the collected descriptive adjectives easier, the GR-SFMPQ is presented in Figure 1.

What makes the McGill Pain Questionnaire, in both its long and short form, a useful tool in the analysis of our data, is that the descriptive words it comprises, though designed to be implemented by health care professionals as part of medical practices, are not purely technical terms, but rather quite familiar lexical forms deriving from everyday experience. As Halliday (1998: 13) notes about such a recognised listing of pain types used by doctors (without, however, specifically referring to the MPQ), "it is of particular interest because it lies at the intersection of the technical register of medical practice with non-technical register of the everyday discussion of personal ailments." The existence of a Greek version of this assessment device has enabled me to gain insights into the qualitative differences of pain properties and has served as a basis for the analysis and categorisation of the descriptors provided by clinicians and patients in the dialogues.

7. As Fernandez and Towery (1996) report, it has been argued (e.g. in the multi-axial IASP Pain Taxonomy, Merskey, 1986) that the subcategories of temporal and spatial are really dimensions of pain, rather than classes of pain descriptors. This conforms to our analysis of pain in terms of seven semantic features among which duration and location are included.

Pain Assessment Questionnaire

Greek term / Gloss / Original English term	No pain Mild Moderate Severe
Sensory descriptors	
palmikos – riθmikos / 'pulsing – rythmic' / throbbing	0)____ 1)____ 2)____ 3)____
san na perpatai / 'as if it walked' / shooting	0)____ 1)____ 2)____ 3)____
san maxeria / 'like a stab' / stabbing	0)____ 1)____ 2)____ 3)____
oksis / 'sharp' / sharp	0)____ 1)____ 2)____ 3)____
san krampa / 'like a cramp' / cramping	0)____ 1)____ 2)____ 3)____
san na δangoni / 'as if it bit' / gnawing	0)____ 1)____ 2)____ 3)____
kafstikos – zestos / 'caustic – hot' / hot – burning	0)____ 1)____ 2)____ 3)____
jenikos – δiarkis / 'general – constant' / aching	0)____ 1)____ 2)____ 3)____
esθima varus / 'sensation of heaviness' / heavy	0)____ 1)____ 2)____ 3)____
evesθitos / 'delicate' / tender	0)____ 1)____ 2)____ 3)____
δjamelistikos – san na se skizi / 'splitting – as if it tore you' / splitting	0)____ 1)____ 2)____ 3)____
Affective descriptors	
kurastikos / 'tiring' / tiring – exhausting	0)____ 1)____ 2)____ 3)____
aiδjastikos – nosiros / 'disgusting – morbid' / sickening	0)____ 1)____ 2)____ 3)____
tromaktikos / 'frightful' / fearful	0)____ 1)____ 2)____ 3)____
vasanistikos – skliros / 'torturing – cruel'/ punishing – cruel	0)____ 1)____ 2)____ 3)____

Present Pain Index (PPI)

1. ipios	(mild)	________
2. enoxlitikos	(discomforting)	________
3. oδiniros	(distressing)	________
4. friktos	(horrible)	________
5. aforitos	(excruciating)	________

Figure 1 Greek version of the short-form McGill Pain Questionnaire (GR-SFMPQ)

7.2.6.1 *The intensity of pain*

Measuring the intensity of pain is one of the most difficult aspects of pain assessment, given that pain is a subjective, private experience, and, therefore, there cannot be any reliably objective pain measurements (see Borsook, LeBel and McPeek, 1998 and DeSouza and Frank, 2000, among others). Consequently, it is only by patients themselves in terms of self-rating scales – constructed in a visual, numerical, verbal or combined form – that intensity can be measured.

Pain intensity is grammatically realised in Greek by an adjective, which may function either as Epithet (e.g. *δinatos ponos* 'strong pain') or Attribute (e.g. *jinan aforiti i poni* 'the pains became unbearable' (or 'excruciating' to use Georgoudis's mapping of *aforitos*). Not only do different types of pain vary in intensity, but also the intensity of a particular pain may fluctuate, e.g. (34). The adjectives denoting degree of intensity that were collected in the Greek data are *liγos* 'little', *metrios* 'moderate', *endonos* 'intense' / 'severe', *δinatos* 'strong', *ipervolikos* 'excessive', e.g. (35), *mejistos* 'greatest', *frixtos* 'horrible', *anektos* 'tolerable', as well as a number of deverbal adjectives ending in *-tos* and prefixed with the negative affix *a-*, which express impossibility of becoming the object of the action denoted by the verb, i.e. impossibility of being V-en: *aδiorθotos* 'irremediable', *avastaxtos* 'intolerable', and *aforitos* 'unbearable'. By far the most frequently observed adjective denoting pain intensity in the doctor-patient dialogues is the affective term *aforitos* 'unbearable', followed by *endonos* 'intense' / 'severe' and *δinatos* 'strong'.[8] Interestingly, only less than half of the adjectives observed actually figure as intensity terms in the GR-SFMPQ on either of the two self-rating scales, namely, *metrios* 'moderate', *endonos* 'intense' / 'severe', *frixtos* 'horrible', and *aforitos* 'unbearable' but not its near-synomym *avastaxtos* 'intolerable'.

(34) D: ne, ala *exi δjakimansis* o ponos, pote iste kala, pote ponate, ap' oti katalaveno.
yes but have-PRS:3SG fluctuations-ACC the pain-NOM sometimes be-PRS:2PL well sometimes hurt-PRS:2PL from what understand-PRS:1SG
'Yes, but the pain *fluctuates*, at times you are well, at times you hurt, from what I understand.'

(35) P: …apo ki ke pera arxinai o ponos.
from there and on start-PRS:3SG the pain-NOM
'…from then on the pain starts.'
D: ne.
yes
'Yes.'
P: ponos *ipervolikos*. δen vastiete me kamia δinami.
pain-NOM excessive-NOM not tolerate-PASS:PRS:3SG with not-any force-ACC
'*Excessive* pain. It can by no means be tolerated.'

There are three more idiosyncratic construals of pain intensity, one in the idiomatic expression *skiloponos*, which is a compound formed from the nouns *skilos* 'dog' and *ponos* 'pain' (literally 'dog-pain'), another in the 'loose appositional compound' *trela pono* 'pain like madness' (literally 'madness-pain') observed in utterance (36), and finally, in the sequence *ponos ponos* 'real pain' (literally 'pain-pain'), the last

8. It is worth noting that, from an initial analysis of *ponos* collocates observed in the pain corpus and the non-specialised Corpus of Greek Texts (CGT) (see note 3 above) that I am currently working on, these three adjectives appear to be the most frequent pain descriptors in the CGT as well, but in a different rank order: it is *endonos* 'intense' / 'severe' which is by far the most frequent, followed by *aforitos* 'unbearable' and *δinatos* 'strong'.

two used to refer to extreme, excruciating pain.[9] (Madness / insanity as a source domain for the metaphorical understanding of pain will be discussed in more detail in Chapter 8. Also, compare *pain is pain is pain*, reported by DeSouza and Frank, 2000: 217, as an expression of amount of pain in terms of its seriousness.) Finally, some doctors used a ten-point rating scale to inquire about pain intensity, e.g. as exemplified in (37).

(36) P: molis sikonome, tak, θeli… kseris ti pono! *trela pono*!
as-soon-as get-up-PRS:1SG tack want-PRS:3SG know-PRS:2SG what pain-ACC madness-ACC pain-ACC
'As soon as I get up, there it is again, it wants… you know what kind of pain! *Pain like madness*!'

(37) D: o vaθmos tu ponu aftu poso ine, an leγame oti *o aforitos* ine 10, *o metrios* ine 5, *o kaθolu* ine 0, esis ti vaθmo…?
the grade-NOM the pain-GEN this-GEN how-much be-PRS:3SG if say-IPFV:1PL that the unbearable-NOM be-PRS:3SG 10 the moderate-NOM be-PRS:3SG 5 the null be-PRS:3SG 0 you-NOM:PL what grade-ACC
'How would you grade this pain, if we said that *unbearable pain* is 10, *moderate pain* is 5, and *no pain* is 0, what grade would you…?'

P: e tora telefteos itane 9.
eh now lately be-IPFV:3SG 9
'Eh, it has been 9 lately.'

9. The construction *ponos trela* (NOM) is a typical example of an increasing number of Greek 'loose appositional compounds', i.e. constructions where a noun modifies the head noun after which it is placed (see Holton, Mackridge and Philippaki-Warburton, 1997: 344–345). Some of the more traditional fixed combinations, e.g. *θalasa laδi* 'smooth sea' (lit. 'sea oil'), *skotaδi pisa* 'pitch dark', are normally used with the appropriate form of the copula verb *ime* 'to be', but can also occur on their own to serve an exclamatory function. While the traditional expressions are typically written as two separate words, there is a tendency for the more recent patterns to be hyphenated: *episkepsi-astrapi* 'lightning visit', *peδi-θavma* 'infant prodigy', *jineka-araxni* 'spider woman'. In most appositional constructions of this type and certainly in all the examples cited here, the second noun (*trela, laδi, pisa, astrapi, θavma, araxni*) serves as the source domain for the metaphorical representation of the first noun (*ponos, θalasa, skotaδi, episkepsi, peδi, jineka*). The observed construction *ponos trela* has an exclamatory function in (36) and appears with a reversal in the order of the two nouns which can be attributed to emphatic reasons: the source domain noun *trela* is preposed by virtue of its focalisation and the accompanying emphatic stress it carries. (See also Nakas and Gavriilidou, 2005.)

7.2.6.2 *The variable qualities of pain*

Pain intensity alone is not, however, a sufficient descriptive dimension. Of crucial importance in the description and assessment of pain in human subjects are its variable qualities. As Melzack and Torgerson (1971: 50) argue, "To describe pain solely in terms of intensity [...] is like specifying the visual world in terms of light flux only, without regard to pattern, color, texture, and many other dimensions of visual experience." In other words, if the endless variety of pain qualities were not specified, it would seem that the single linguistic label *ponos* (*pain* in English and their translation equivalents in other languages), under which they are categorised, referred to a particular sensation that could only vary in intensity. This would mean that the pains of e.g. a broken leg, a scalded hand, angina pectoris, arthritis, ulcerative colitis, as well as earaches, migraine, and labour pains, could not be qualitatively differentiated from one another but, rather, would constitute a single quality experience, distinguishable in terms of intensity only. However, medical practices, everyday experience, and the multitude of words used to describe this experiential domain undoubtedly show that this is not the case. In actual fact, despite their diversity and multitude, our arbitrary and conventional, i.e. symbolic, linguistic labels used for classes and subclasses of pain turn out to be too restricted and narrow compared to our pain experiences (see Melzack and Torgerson, *ibid.*).

An examination of the GR-SFMPQ reveals that the majority of sensory qualities are linguistically realised by means of metaphorically structured adjectives or adjectival participles in English, whereas in Greek, their translation into corresponding adjectival forms not always being possible, periphrastic *san* 'like' + noun / verb, i.e. 'as if' expressions are resorted to. In both languages, however, the descriptors have an analogy 'as if' meaning, i.e. they are figures of speech whereby, by virtue of a particular quality, the pain sensation is likened to the mode of (or the instrument / means used in) an unpleasant, harmful, or aggressive action potentially producing injury or pain. Thus, for example, the term *stabbing* and its Greek translation *san maxeria* are not intended to literally refer to a sensation caused by actual stabbing but, rather, to a sensation that the patient could imagine to approximate to (be as if) one evoked by stabbing. (For a discussion of simile, identifiable by the use of the word *like*, as a common means whereby subjects provide graphic descriptions of the quality of their experienced pain, see DeSouza and Frank, 2000: 212, and Melzack and Torgerson, 1971: 58). As Fernandez and Towery (1996: 32) point out, unless metaphorically understood, "the word *stabbing*... would have little if any place in the vocabulary of a pain patient who had never been stabbed before." In fact, for some of the most extreme categories of pain, such as *splitting* in *splitting headache*, or *shooting* and *stabbing*, it is, obviously, rather unlikely that the patient providing the descriptor could ever have undergone an actual related experience. (For an analysis of *burning* and *splitting*, see Melzack and

Torgerson, *ibid.*: 58. Also for a discussion of *flickering* and *boring*, see Fernandez and Towery, 1996: 32.) To conclude, by means of sensory pain descriptors, the various qualities of the pain sensation are metaphorically represented in terms of a range of metonymically derived (physical) causes, the general metonymic relationship INSTRUMENT / MEANS FOR ACTION / EVENT forming their metonymic basis. (See Chapter 8, section 8.2.3 for an extensive discussion of the conceptual mechanisms (metonymies and metaphors) involved in the understanding of the various types of (actual or potential) tissue damage causing different types of painful sensation, where it is suggested that these cognitive processes are also constrained by universal aspects of human physiology, potentially giving rise to similar linguistic realisations across languages.)

The metaphorical structuring of sensory pain descriptors is also put forward by Fabrega and Tyma (1976b: 354). (For the role of metaphorical expressions in descriptions of the sensory qualities of pain provided by fibromyalgia patients, see Söderberg and Norberg, 1995 and Hallberg and Carlsson, 2000.) They argue that what they classify as *secondary pain terms*,[10] i.e. words which denote physical change of state or damage, "are employed as qualifying metaphors in pain description (as in 'I have a *crushing* pain')", i.e. these terms refer to "what the perceptual experience of pain is being likened to." They suggest that such pain terms as *burning, cutting, crushing*, etc. are critically involved in the elaboration of the pain experience, a "negative or injurious physical change of a seemingly equally physical object" certainly embracing them semantically (*ibid.*: 365). Hence, they suggest, this type of damage seems to constitute significant source domains for the metaphorical description of pain. Consequently, key semantic features of pain should be revealed if these terms are analysed and a version or model of what pain is or stands for in a particular language (and culture) should emerge. Thus, according to Fabrega and Tyma (*ibid.*: 364), "the 'model' for pain descriptions in English [...] has a physical basis, suggesting that the experience itself has and is being likened to a physical process." Their central argument is that an important factor motivating the metaphorical aspects of pain descriptions is to be sought in the impossibility of assigning precision – by virtue of validation effected through direct and con-

10. Fabrega and Tyma (1976b) identify three classes of terms used in utterances of pain description. In addition to *secondary pain terms* discussed here, they formulate *primary pain terms*, i.e. a limited number of words, such as 'pain', 'ache', 'hurt', and 'sore', which serve as a base for the description of the perceptual experience which they define as pain, and *tertiary pain terms*, i.e. terms of qualification that are used to register degree of intensity, fullness, duration, and so on ('I have an *intense* pain in my leg'). Moreover, they also include under the category of tertiary pain terms those which refer to body parts, such as back, leg, stomach, etc. as they explicitly link the pain experience to the body, this linkage to the body representing a necessary feature of pain as defined in their study.

sensual observation – to perceptual experiences arising entirely from within the body, as is the case with words used to describe concrete objects (e.g. tree, sun, car, etc.). Our data analysis suggests that this assumption could plausibly be extended to Greek (secondary, sensory) pain terms and that an observable, natural and physical process "captured by deformation, destruction, damage and harm" (*ibid.*: 364) is also implicated. Interestingly, Söderberg and Norberg (1995) also refer to Fabrega and Tyma's (1976b) assumption of a physical model on which English pain language is often based and suggest a similar model of pain (as an aggressive physical deformation and a torture-like experience) underlying Swedish pain expressions as it emerges from their interviews with fibromyalgia patients.

Turning now to our Greek doctor-patient data, the observed descriptive adjectives used to specify pain qualities are: the sensory descriptors *kinitos* 'moving', *δiaxitos* 'diffused', *leptos* 'fine', *anepesθitos* 'imperceptible', *vaθis* 'deep', *ylikos* 'sweet', e.g. (38), *mundos* 'dull', *kseros* 'dry', *oksis* / *oksitatos* 'sharp' / 'sharpest', and the affective words *viosimos* 'viable', *aljotikos* 'distinct', *tromeros* 'fearful', *sovaros* 'serious', and *oxi astios* 'not funny'. There is also an instance of the affective adjective *alipitos* 'merciless' / 'unpitying', whereby pain is configured as the subject rather than the object of the verb from which this form is derived, and is, thus, allowed to be metaphorically construed as a cruel animate entity. In addition, three medical, technical terms occurred, namely, *zostiroiδis* 'zoster-like', *mioskeletikos* 'musculoskeletal', and *miikos* 'muscular', while the term *revmatikos* 'rheumatic' was used as part of a simile, i.e. *san revmatikos ponos* 'like rheumatic pain'. There is also an instance of the periphrastic expression *ponos se suvlies* 'piercing pain' in (45) below.

(38) P: δen ponai akrivos, ine *ylikos* ponos.
not hurt-PRS:IMPERS:3SG exactly be-PRS:3SG sweet pain-NOM
'It doesn't hurt really, it's a *sweet* pain.'

The questions most commonly used by medical experts to probe pain qualities in the material are:

(39) *ti ponos* ine aftos?
what pain-NOM be-PRS:3SG this-NOM
'*What (kind of) pain* is this?'

(40) *pos ine* aftos o ponos?
how be-PRS:3SG this the pain-NOM
'*How does* this pain *feel*?'

Sometimes the doctor invites the patient to describe the qualities of his pain by comparing it to something else that he (the doctor) either leaves unspecified, e.g. (41) and (45) or refers to by means of explicit metaphorically structured clues, e.g.

(42), (43), and (45). Hence, the medical expert may not only encourage the sufferer to talk about his painful sensation in metaphorical terms, but he may also provide the patient with the conceptual source domain from which he can structure his experiential target domain, i.e. his pain, in more familiar and concrete terms. Therefore, metaphorical descriptors are either spontaneously supplied by the patient, as in (44), or they are elicited by the health professional, as in (42), (43), and (45). Consider the following passages from the dialogues:

(41) D: *ti ponos* in' aftos? *pos ine? pos, san ti miazi* aftos o ponos?
what pain-NOM be-PRS:3SG this-NOM how be-PRS:3SG how like what-ACC resemble-PRS:3SG this the pain-NOM
'*What (kind of) pain* is this? *What is it like? How, what does* this pain *resemble?*'

(42) D: o ponos aftos *pos ine? san na sas pernai revma?*
the pain-NOM this-NOM how be-PRS:3SG like to-PARTCL you-ACC pass-PRS:3SG current-NOM
'*How does* this pain *feel? As if a flow of electricity is passing through you?*'

(43) D: *ti iδus* ponos ine? *suvlia, maxeria, sfiksimo, varis, sfiri, tsekuri?*
what kind-GEN pain-NOM be-PRS:3SG piercing-NOM stab-NOM squeezing-NOM heavy-NOM hammer-NOM hatchet-NOM
'*What kind of pain* is this? *Piercing, like a stab, squeezing, heavy, like a hammer, a hatchet?*'

(44) P: o ponos ine *aforitos…* ine ee *san na ine ena sirma* apo mesa ke *strivi*, etsi to esθanome.
the pain-NOM be-PRS:3SG unbearable-NOM be-PRS:3SG hmhm like to-PARTCL be-PRS:3SG a wire-NOM from inside and turn-around-PRS:3SG like-this it-ACC feel-PRS:1SG
'The pain is *unbearable…* It is *as if there is a wire* inside *which is turning around*, that's how I feel it.'

(45) D: *ti xaraktira exi aftos o ponos? pos in' aftos o ponos?*
what character-ACC have-PRS:3SG this the pain-NOM how be-PRS:3SG this the pain-NOM
'*What is the character of this pain? How does this pain feel?*'

P: ine *ponos se suvlies.*
be-PRS:3SG pain-NOM in piercing-ACC
'It's *a piercing pain.*'

D: ne, ine *san na sas tripai kapjos me maxeri*, ine kapos *san revma na pernai…*
yes be-PRS:3SG like to-PARTCL you-ACC pierce-PRS:3SG someone-NOM with knife-ACC be-PRS:3SG somewhat like current-NOM to-PARTCL pass-PRS:3SG
'Yes, it's *as if someone is piercing you with a knife*, it's somewhat *like a flow of electricity is passing through you*.'

P: *suvlies.*
piercing-NOM
'*Piercing pains*.'

D: *suvlies… suvlies.*
piercing piercing-NOM
'*Piercing pains… piercing pains*.'

P: *suvlies, suvlies, erxete* o ponos *fevji, ksanarxete* ke sta δio γonata.
piercing piercing-NOM come-PRS:3SG the pain-NOM go-PRS:3SG come-back-PRS:3SG and in-the two knees-ACC
'*Piercing, piercing*, the pain *comes and goes, it comes back* in both knees.'

The complexity of the pain experience is reflected in the fact that despite the reliability and validity of the SFMPQ in both its original English version and the Greek one, the pain descriptors observed in our authentic doctor-patient dialogues, cannot easily be mapped onto those of the questionnaire. Surprisingly, of the collected adjectives denoting pain quality, only *oksis* 'sharp' appears in the GR-SFMPQ, while the observed *tromeros* 'fearful' is very close to, though not as strong as, *tromaktikos* 'frightful', which, however, figures as the Greek translation equivalent of the original English *fearful*. Of the remaining descriptors, *kinitos* 'moving' corresponds to *san na perpatai* 'as if it walked', but cannot be equated to the original English *shooting*, while *δiaxitos* 'diffused', which also reflects spatial properties of pain, cannot be related to any of the questionnaire terms, unless interpreted along a temporal dimension, in which case it could be seen as related to *jenikos – δiarkis* 'general – constant' *aching*. Moreover, *leptos* 'fine', if interpreted as 'sharp' rather than 'delicate', corresponds to *oksis*, while *anepesθitos* 'imperceptible' could be compared to *evesθitos* 'delicate' *tender*. The affective adjective *viosimos* 'viable' could perhaps be understood as the negative equivalent of either *kurastikos* 'tiring' *tiring – exhausting* or *vasanistikos – skliros* 'torturing – cruel' *punishing – cruel*, unless interpreted as an antonym of *aforitos* 'unbearable' *excruciating*, which is an intensity rather than a quality term. On the grounds that *alipitos* 'merciless' / 'unpitying' denotes an entity lacking in mercy and pity, it can be mapped onto the strongest affective term in the questionnaire, i.e. *vasanistikos – skliros* 'torturing – cruel' *punishing – cruel*. The negatively construed affective descriptor *oxi astios* 'not funny' could also be related to *vasanistikos – skliros* 'torturing – cruel' *punish-*

ing – *cruel*, if interpreted as deriving from the idiomatic expression *δen astievete* '(s)he is not joking', i.e. '(s)he is merciless / unpitying'. As for the sensory descriptors *vaθis* 'deep', *mundos* 'dull', *kseros* 'dry', and *γlikos* 'sweet', and the affective ones *aljotikos* 'distinct' and *sovaros* 'serious' there do not seem to be terms in the GR-SFMPQ to which they can be closely associated, though *dull* figures in the original English long version of the MPQ.

To conclude, the variety of observed quality descriptive adjectives and the difficulty of mapping them onto the GR-SFMPQ terms indicate that it is extremely difficult, if not impossible, to devise exhaustive lists of pain descriptors so as to classify types of pain. It appears that new pain categories and new members of the categories can actually result from everyday experience and medical practice, i.e. they do not constitute 'a closed system' (see also Halliday, 1998: 13). It seems that the need to communicate pain – in terms of intensity, quality, and affective reaction – is so strong on the part of the patients that they may become quite creative and innovative with respect to the descriptors they employ, often resorting to less conventional or predictable terms, e.g. the metaphorically structured affective descriptors *alipitos* 'merciless' / 'unpitying' or *oxi astios* 'not funny' observed in the Greek doctor-patient data. An interesting example is also provided by DeSouza and Frank (2000: 216) who report in their study that individuals experiencing chronic back pain used a wider range of descriptors in their 'insider' accounts than the MPQ would have allowed them to do, expressing their pain as visual (*red*) and auditory (*shouting*) sensations. Besides, some of the MPQ terms may be incomprehensible to the majority of patients, e.g. the English words *lancinating* and *rasping* or the Greek word *δjamelistikos* 'splitting' and, therefore, it is quite improbable that they will be spontaneously used by patients. On the other hand, Fernandez and Towery (1996: 32) maintain that it is quite likely that "the (universal) vocabulary of pain is smaller than that suggested in the MPQ," given that the number of descriptors included in the original English version has been substantially reduced in many of its translations and adaptations.

7.2.7 Concluding remarks

The evidence derived from the Greek corpus data clearly suggests that it is by means of its diverse qualities that this domain of human experience is essentially identified and qualified: the other pain features are not exclusively associated with pain, though they may significantly contribute to the identification and assessment of the painful experience. In Fabrega and Tyma's (1976b: 363–364) understanding, pain terms denoting qualities formulated as physical change of state or damage "realize criterial features of pain," while terms of qualification that are used to register degree of intensity, fullness, duration, and so on (i.e. *tertiary pain terms*) do not bear special connection to pain *per se*. Instead, these terms appear to be used purely to qualify any experience, their importance being precisely that they refer to general attributes of many types of phenomena. Fabrega and Tyma propose that "the English version of pain," despite its unique features, "is not totally unique in that it shares parameters common to other 'objects' in the language (e.g. emotions) and by implication is registered like other mental and physical phenomena." However, they argue, this should not necessarily be considered a universal feature of pain.

To conclude, my data-based lexico-grammatical analysis of *ponos* in terms of the seven grammatically construed semantic features of pain proposed by Halliday (1998) (bounded or unbounded entity, possession, temporal location and extent, accompanying conditions, location within the body, variable intensity, and variable qualities) has shown that these features are dimensions along which pain may be reported and made an 'object' in Greek. Hence, when lexically realised as the noun *ponos*, pain lends itself to being described, measured and assessed. That such descriptive utterances, where pain is construed as a participant in a process rather than the process itself, belong to the descriptive pole of our proposed integrating continuum of pain manifestations will be further supported in our subsequent discussion of *ponos* nominal constructions.

7.3 Structural configurations featuring *ponos* as participant

We shall now examine each one of the structural configurations into which *ponos* enters as a participant. Appendix B presents both the Greek patterns derived from our doctor-patient material and Halliday's English paradigm of pain as 'thing'. The Greek constructions and their corresponding English ones will be referred to by means of their numbering in that paradigm. Representative examples drawn from the corpus will be used to illustrate our discussion.

Unlike what was done in our presentation of pain as process, in our examination of *ponos* nominal constructions we shall not be concerned with frequency counts. The reason is that the noun *ponos* was found to occur not only as a participant in processes realised by 'full' clauses but also quite frequently in elliptical ones, in false starts, in 'echo' structures, or in constructions involving repetition. In other words there is no one-to-one correspondence between the number of *ponos* occurrences and the number of clauses where it functions as a process participant. Hence, it was considered unnecessarily cumbersome to attempt any calculation of the actual 'participant' occurrences of *ponos* in frequency terms. Instead it was judged appropriate to restrict our discussion to the analysis of the structural configurations in terms of process type and structural functions and simply refer to very gross frequency considerations.

(46) ***exo (enan) pono sti mesi*** No 15 of the paradigm
have-PRS:1SG pain-ACC in-the low-back-ACC
'I've got (a) pain in the / my low back'

The configuration *exo (enan) pono sti mesi*, which occurred most frequently in the material, is a relational process of the possessive type and attributive mode, i.e. one in which a relation of possession is established between two entities, here the sufferer and pain (similarly, *exo (ena) sinaxi* 'I've got a cold in the head'). In this pattern the relation of possession is encoded as the Process with the possessor-sufferer configured as the Carrier of the Attribute, i.e. of the possessed-pain. Thus, pain-possession is an attribute ascribed to the sufferer. Unlike English, where the possessor as Carrier is linguistically expressed by means of a separate (pronominal) constituent, in Greek, as has already been noted, due to the fact that personal pronoun subjects are suppressed unless emphatic or contrastive, the Carrier is linguistically realised through the suffix of the verb *exo*. Utterances (47)-(50) are typical examples of this possessive configuration:

(47) P: *ixa enan endono pono s' afto to simio…*
have-PST:1SG an intense pain-ACC in this the spot-ACC
'*I had an intense pain in this spot…*'

(48) D: ap' oti vlepo, *δen ixate pote oksi pono…*
from what see-PRS:1SG not have-PST:2PL never sharp pain-ACC
'From what I can see, *you've never had sharp pain…*'

(49) P: eno sto xorio… *ixa δinatus ponus* ke ti nixta akomi.
whereas at-the village-ACC have-PST:1SG strong pains-ACC and the night-ACC even
'Whereas at my village… even at night *I had strong pains*.'

(50) D: *ixate ponus ston afxena* tote?
have-PST:2PL pains-ACC in-the neck-ACC then
'*Did you have any pains in the neck* at that time?'

However, as was pointed out when we discussed the semantic feature of possession in relation to *ponos* in section 7.2, this is not a typical possessive relationship (cf. *o angelos exi teseris kiθares* 'Angelos has four guitars'). We shall be able to reach a more subtle and solid interpretation of *exo + ponos* patterns in Chapter 8, section 8.2.1, when we examine the combined effect of the syntactico-semantic features of *exo* and *ponos* in determining the understanding of such pain expressions. Hence, it will be argued that *exo + ponos* constructions are understood as predominantly possessive processes by virtue of (a) the interpretation of *exo* as primarily a possessive rather than a semantically empty linking (i.e. delexical) verb in such patterns, this semantic analysis being motivated by (b) the prevalent construal of *ponos* as profiling a particular instance of the painful experience rather than a type of feeling when it co-occurs with *exo*.

Moreover, in the investigation of the conceptual basis of pain language to be presented in Chapter 8, possessive *exo* + *ponos* constructions will be shown to have a central role in the metaphorical representation of pain. What is more, their interpretation from a cognitive semantic perspective will provide a justification for the insights expressed by Halliday from his functional perspective.

In particular, it will be argued that the source domain POSSESSION OF AN OBJECT is applied to express the 'existence' of pain (e.g. *exo* ena fovero *ponokefalo* 'I *have* a terrible *headache*'), hence the metaphor EXISTENCE OF PAIN IS POSSESSION OF AN OBJECT / A POSSESSED OBJECT, in much the same way as it is applied to conceptualise the existence of an emotion, i.e. in the metaphor EXISTENCE OF EMOTION IS POSSESSION OF AN OBJECT / A POSSESSED OBJECT (e.g. *exume* mja meγali *stenoxoria* 'we *have* a great *sadness*'). It is noteworthy that the concepts of 'attribution' and 'possession', also invoked in Halliday's functional analysis presented above, play an equally essential part in the instantiation of this metaphor, schematically represented as follows: a state (e.g. an emotional state, such as pain) can be understood as an attribute, and attributes are conceptualised as possessed objects (that may be given, acquired, owned, preserved, and lost). Hence, the metaphor (EXISTENCE OF) PAIN IS A POSSESSION / A POSSESSED OBJECT emerges as an instantiation of the higher-level metaphor ATTRIBUTES ARE POSSESSED OBJECTS.

The analysis of *exo* + *ponos* metaphorical representations of pain to be presented in the next chapter will provide a cognitive semantic interpretation for their functional account presented in this chapter. I suggest, therefore, that the two accounts complement each other in a very attractive way, by virtue of the existence of a significant degree of correspondence between the two approaches as regards the metaphorical understanding of human experience. It is actually the fact that such seemingly dissimilar linguistic approaches reveal this degree of convergence that makes their juxtaposition so appealing.

(51) ***afto mu δini / ferni / prokali / kani ponokefalo*** — Nos 16 & 17 of the paradigm
this-NOM I-GEN give / bring / cause / make-PRS:3SG headache-ACC
'That gives / is giving me a headache'

As has already been mentioned in our discussion of pain as process (Chapter 6, section 6.3), the absence of a simple present – present continuous morphological distinction in Greek, parallel to the one that exists in English, makes it necessary to rely on the context in order to interpret certain utterances with respect to their time reference. This is also the case with the structure *afto mu δini / ferni / prokali / kani ponokefalo*, which corresponds to two English configurations provided by Halliday in his paradigm.

More specifically, when interpreted as corresponding to *that gives me a headache*, this structure may be understood as relational: attributive of the possessive agentive type, *afto* (an object or process) being configured as the Agent. Hence, it may be understood as the agentive agnate of the relational: attributive / possessive structure (15) *exo pono sti mesi* 'I've got (a) pain in the / my low back'. On the other hand, when this construction is related to *that's giving me a headache*, it is interpreted as a process of 'doing' involving an Actor and a Goal, i.e. a material process typically having a clear beginning and ending. In this construal, the sufferer is configured as Beneficiary, i.e. the entity that is 'given' the pain (Goal) caused by another non-conscious entity or process. With this interpretation, it could be compared to the two-participant material: effective construction (12) *afto me ponai* 'that's hurting me', where the Actor is again another, non-conscious, entity but the Goal is the sufferer rather than the painful sensation, the latter being lexicalised through the verb itself. Surprisingly, this *ponos* construction, in both its interpretations, occurred quite marginally in the data. Such constructions as *afto mu ferni ipno / nista* 'that makes / is making me sleepy', *afto mu δini xara / efxaristisi* 'that gives / is giving me joy / pleasure' or *afto mu prokali meγali θlipsi / ekpliksi* 'that causes / is causing great sorrow / surprise to me', can be seen as the closest agnates of the above *ponos* configuration. The data under (52) and (53) contain instances of this *ponos* construal.

(52) P: δen ksero *ti mu prokali tus ponus.*
not know-PRS:1SG what I-GEN cause-PRS:3SG the pains-ACC
'I don't know *what it is that causes me the pains.*'

(53) P: palia me esfinge, me esfinge ala *mu eδine* ke tin teliki…
before I-ACC squeeze-IPFV:3SG I-ACC squeeze-IPFV:3SG but I-GEN give-IPFV:3SG and the final-ACC
'It used to squeeze me, to squeeze me but *it* also *gave me* the final…'

D: aaaa.
ah
'Ah.'

P: …*ton teliko pono.*
the final pain-ACC
'…*the final pain.*'

D: aaaa. ne.
ah yes
'Ah, yes.'

P: eno *δen mu ton δini.*
whereas not I-GEN it-ACC give-PRS:3SG
'Whereas *it doesn't give it to me* (any more).'

(54) ***njoθis eki pono***? No 18 of the paradigm
feel-PRS:2SG there pain-ACC
'Do you feel any pain there?'

In *njoθo* 'I feel' + *ponos* configurations the sufferer and his pain are the two participants in a mental process, one of perception, in particular. They typically involve a Senser, the conscious being that is sensing, here the sufferer, and a Phenomenon, i.e. that which is sensed, here the painful experience (cf. other perception clauses, e.g. *akus θorivo*? 'do you hear (any) noise?', *vlepis fos*? 'do you see (any) light?'). In addition to the verb *njoθo*, its synonym *esθanome* also occurred in the data. Like *exo* + *ponos* possessive clauses, where pain is understood as possessed Attribute, this construction, where pain is construed as the syntactic object of a transitive verb denoting perception, will prove to be of central importance in paving the way for our account of metaphorically structured *ponos* configurations. In (55) and (56) the verb *esθanome* co-occurs with the bare singular form of *ponos* realising its construal as an unbounded thing, which, as we shall see in our discussion of the metaphorical structuring of *ponos*, is typical of *esθanome* / *njoθo* + *ponos* patterns.

(55) D: *esθaneste pono* i δisaresto sinesθima?
feel-PRS:2PL pain-ACC or unpleasant sensation-ACC
'*Do you feel pain* or discomfort?'

(56) P: *esθanome* ke pali *pono* eδo mesa.
feel-PRS:1SG and again pain-ACC in here
'Once more *I feel pain* in here.'

(57) ***o ponos mu ine avastaxtos ti nixta*** No 19 of the paradigm
the pain-NOM my be-PRS:3SG
intolerable-NOM the night-ACC
'My pain is intolerable at night.'

This type of clause and *exo pono* constructions were found to be the two most frequently occurring in the doctor-patient dialogues. It is a typical relational attributive process, whereby a multitude of properties may be assigned to the painful experience, which functions as the Carrier. This is in fact a construction very commonly used by both doctors and patients to specify or inquire about the degree of intensity and the various qualities of pain. In this configuration, therefore, pain is understood as an entity that can be identified and described in terms of related qualitative and quantitative features (cf. *i elpiδes mu ine lijes* 'my hopes are few', *i ayonia mu ine meyali* 'my agony is great'). Consequently, the painful sensation is essentially construed as an element that lends itself to being objectified. Consider the following:

(58) P: …*o* telefteos *ponos itane* pjo *endonos*.
the last pain-NOM be-PST:3SG more intense-NOM
'…*the* last *pain was* more *intense*.'

(59) P: *kseros ine o ponos* s' afto to simio.
dry-NOM be-PRS:3SG the pain-NOM in this the spot-ACC
'*The pain is dry* in this spot.'

(60) P: *ine viosimos* ja mena *o ponos… anektos* ja mena.
be-PRS:3SG viable-NOM for I-ACC the pain-NOM tolerable-NOM for I-ACC
'For me *the pain is viable… tolerable*.'

(61) ***to 10 ine o aforitos ponos*** No 22 of the paradigm
the 10 be-PRS:3SG the excruciating pain-NOM
'Score 10 is / represents the excruciating pain'

The pattern *to 10 ine o aforitos ponos* is one of the two Greek structures observed in the corpus that do not correspond to any of the pain expressions featuring in Halliday's paradigm of pain as 'thing'. Here *ponos* is the Carrier in a relational process where an identity rather than some quality is assigned to it. Thus, a numerical score functioning as Identifier / Token is used to identify pain construed as the Identified / Value, in terms of its intensity (cf. *o vaθmos 20 ine to "arista"* 'grade 20 is "excellent"'). It is by virtue of the reversibility of identifying clauses that the function of Identified is ascribed to *ponos* rather than to the score, despite the fact that the former does not bear the syntactic function of subject, typically associated with Identified. Sentence (62) further exemplifies this structure:

(62) D: *10 ine o mejistos ponos, o aforitos.*
10 be-PRS:3SG the greatest pain-NOM the excruciating-NOM
'*(Score) 10 is the greatest pain, the excruciating one*.'

(63) ***ine enas ponos eδo*** No 23 of the paradigm
be-PRS:3SG a pain-NOM here
'There is (a) pain here'

Like (61), the construction of the type *ine enas ponos eδo* derived form the Greek data does not have any equivalent in Halliday's account of English patterns. It is an existential: existing clause, one representing that something, which is labelled Existent, simply exists (cf. *ine enas aγnostos sto γrafio* 'there is a stranger in the office'). Pain being the Existent in this configuration, it follows that it is objectified, since, by definition, any entity that is assigned this function is assumed to be construed as a 'thing'. I suggest that this construal of *ponos* is very closely related to the impersonal *ponai* (*eδo*) 'it hurts (here)' already analysed as existential: existing in the discussion of pain as process. Compared to it, however, this *ponos* configuration allows for a finer identification of the sensation in terms of reference to its subtle properties, given that here pain is linguistically realised as a noun. This is clearly observed in the following data derived from our dialogues:

(64) D: *aftos o ponos itan* ke prin tin enxirisi? panda sto iδio meros? sinexja? i...?
this the pain-NOM exist-PST:3SG and before the operation-ACC always in-the same place-ACC continuously or
'*Did this pain also exist* before the operation? Always in the same place? Continuously? Or...?'

P: tora *ine ke apo oles tis meries.*
now be-PRS:3SG and from all the sides-ACC
'Now *it is all over*.'

(65) P: *ine enas ponos eδo* pu poles fores exo tin esθisi oti ine to nefro mu.
exist-PRS:3SG a pain-NOM here that many times-ACC have-PRS:1SG the feeling-ACC that be-PRS:3SG the kidney-NOM my
'*There is a pain here* that I often have the impression it is my kidney.'

Of the remaining two patterns of Halliday's paradigm, namely 20 and 21 in Appendix B, the former has no equivalent in Greek, while the latter, though possible in Greek, was not represented in the corpus.

More specifically, no construction directly corresponding to Halliday's *are you in* (*great*) *pain*?, i.e. one with the verb *ime* 'to be' and *se* 'in' + *ponos*, exists in Greek (e.g. **ise se* (*meγalo*) *pono?*), despite the possibility of agnate expressions of emotions, such as *ime se* (*meγali*) *aγonia* / *anisixia* 'I am in (great) suspense / distress.' There are, however, *se* 'in' + *ponos* circumstantial construals co-occurring with other verbs, such as *trelenome ston pono*, literally 'I'm going crazy in (the) pain', and *peθeno stus ponus*, literally 'I die in (the) pains', where pain is profiled as a circumstance of cause.[11]

In the original English pattern, the prepositional phrase *in pain* is understood as a circumstance of abstract Location, which, according to Halliday (1998: 23), is "typical of the expression of mental states and conditions." Interestingly, as we shall see in the next chapter, within the cognitive semantic approach (e.g. Lakoff, 1990, 1993; Kövecses, 2000) similar linguistic expressions denoting existence of emotions such as *she is in love*, or the Greek patterns *ime se foveri ayonia* 'I am in terrible suspense', *imaste se paniko* 'we are in panic', are understood as instantiations of the very general metaphor EXISTENCE OF EMOTION IS BEING IN A BOUNDED SPACE which applies to all emotion concepts. This source domain, however, is not unique to emotion concepts, i.e. it is part of the way we conceptualise events in general (e.g. states, changes of states, actions, etc.). Hence, in both the functional and the cognitive semantic analysis, the English expressions *are you in (great) pain? / I am in (great) pain* may be interpreted as representing the existence of pain in terms of a space within which the self is located.[12] Moreover, as we shall see in the relevant discussion of Greek metaphorical *ponos* constructions in Chapter 8, this space may take on the additional meaning of a confining space or prison.

(66) ***o ponos ipoδiloni / δixni oti...*** No 21 of the paradigm
the pain-NOM suggest / show-PRS:3SG (that)
'The pain suggests / shows that...'
[*not extracted from the data*]

The pattern *o ponos ipoδiloni / δixni oti...* corresponding to No 21 of Halliday's paradigm did not occur in our Greek dialogues. The original English construction *the pain suggests / shows that...* is interpreted as a verbal clause, i.e. one representing a symbolic process of 'saying', with pain having the function of Sayer. As such processes cover "any kind of symbolic exchange of meaning" (Halliday, 1985/1994:

11. In addition, *ponos* may appear in other circumstantial construals, which will not systematically concern us here, as they deserve to be dealt with thoroughly in a separate survey of *ponos* as circumstance. Some of these were observed in the corpus and will be mentioned below in the analysis of *ponos* metaphorical configurations (Chapter 8), e.g. *apo* 'from' + *ponos* as in *lipoθimisa apo ton pono* 'I fainted from (the) pain', *ksipnao apo tus ponus* 'I wake up from (the) pains', where pain is profiled as a circumstance of cause, or *me* 'with' + *ponos* patterns, where pain functions as a circumstance of accompaniment, e.g. *emaθes na zis me ton pono su* 'you have learnt to live with your pain', *ksipnisa pali me ponus* 'I woke up again with pains'.

12. The analysis of *in pain* as a circumstance of abstract Location within the functional approach and as denoting a bounded space within the cognitive approach, does not mean that the linguistic expression *I am in pain* is actually the answer to the question *where are you emotionally these days?*.

140), their central participant, the Sayer, need not be an entity endowed with consciousness, but rather anything that can be understood as emitting a signal, e.g. *the clock, his fears, her reaction*, etc. Hence, both in the Greek pattern *o ponos ipoδiloni / δixni oti…* and the English one *the pain suggests / shows that…* the painful sensation is symbolically and metaphorically configured as a source of information actively contributing to the understanding of the patient's condition.

7.3.1 Concluding remarks

Summing up the types of 'figure' into which pain as thing enters in the constructions collected in our Greek doctor-patient dialogues, we observe that *ponos* is represented as a 'participant' directly entering into three of Halliday's four primary types of figure, namely, 'doing', e.g. (17), 'sensing', e.g. (18), and 'being and having', e.g. (19), (23), and (15).

What is of crucial importance in our analysis is that, in as many as five out of the seven English patterns put forward by Halliday (1998: 17, 22–23) where the painful sensation is construed as a participant, it is realised syntactically as a non-subject constituent.[13] That is, in only two of his examples is pain the syntactic subject of the clause. These are *my pain is bad today* – to which the Greek *o ponos mu ine avastaxtos ti nixta* (No19 of the paradigm) relates structurally – where it is the subject of a relational: attributive clause functioning as the Carrier of an Attribute, and *the pain suggests* (*that*)… – whose Greek translation equivalent *o ponos ipoδiloni / δixni oti…* (No 21of the paradigm), however, was not observed in the data – where pain is the subject of a transitive verbal rather than material process and is interpreted as the Sayer rather than the Actor. Therefore, despite the fact that pain is the syntactic subject in this last example, it is not construed as 'doing' something to some other entity, i.e. to a Goal. In brief, nowhere in Halliday's paradigm of 'pain as thing' – where his metaphorically structured intuitions are captured – is pain assigned the transitive function of Actor or the ergative function of (external) Agent.

As we shall see in the following chapter, it is only when we depart from these more common and unmarked patterns of pain to other metaphorically structured expressions that we do find configurations where *ponos* is construed as the Actor in processes of 'doing' or 'doing something to some other entity', i.e. syntactically realised as the subject (a) of an intransitive verb (e.g. of motion) or (b) of a transitive one.

13. See Lascaratou and Marmaridou, 2005.

CHAPTER 8

Pain and metaphor

8.1 Introduction

As has been pointed out by Fabrega and Tyma (1976a: 350), in addition to having a linguistic dimension, pain also has an abstract conceptual dimension, i.e. people talk about pain and derive theories to explain it. In this sense, they argue, "pain is similar to any other abstract cultural category which has no visible or material form; for example, disease, loyalty, fear, and/or evilness." Significant evidence for the way patients conceive pain may be derived from the language they use.

The central role of ordinary language in uncovering the conceptualisation or folk understandings, (i.e. shared, structured knowledge, variously called folk theories / models, cultural models, or idealised cognitive models) of human experience, and in particular emotional experiences, is emphasised by Kövecses (2000) in his cognitive linguistic account of the language of emotions. He argues that emotion language provides a complex and rich picture of what human beings consciously feel when they experience an emotion and, therefore, we must seriously consider our language and folk conceptualisations of emotions, if we wish to reach an understanding of our 'conscious feelings'. Most importantly, Kövecses claims that the everyday words and phrases that native speakers of a language commonly use to talk about particular emotional experiences (e.g. anger, fear, happiness, love, etc.) are pervaded by metaphor in English (and in all probability in other languages as well).

In the cognitive linguistic view, metaphor is a cognitive process, whereby aspects of one conceptual domain of experience (usually an abstract, intangible, or complex one, the target domain) are understood in terms of aspects of another conceptual domain (usually a more concrete, tangible, physical, or familiar one, the source domain). When a concept is metaphorically structured, the language used is also metaphorically structured. "So the metaphor is not merely in the words we use – it is in our very concept of an argument" (Lakoff and Johnson, 1981: 289). Therefore, much of our conceptual system being metaphorically understood, the bulk of our everyday conventional language is an important source of evidence for what our conceptual system is like. Moreover, as Gibbs (1999: 40–41) suggests, metaphoric processing is "a general mode of understanding that can be applied to any kind of situation or language": it might legitimately be viewed as one type of cognitive strategy employed by people "as an indispensable part of making sense of many ordinary events in their lives" and of better understanding real-world experiences, just as it may colour their imaginative understanding of texts.

Along these lines, Kövecses (*ibid.*: 191–2) maintains that it is essentially through the mediation of metaphor that emotion language is able to capture the variety of diverse and intangible emotional experiences and to offer an understanding of most aspects of the conceptualisation of emotion. Crucially, he argues, the language does not merely reflect the experiences but it also creates them. In his own words (*ibid.*: 192), "Simply put, we say what we feel and we feel what we say."

The view that metaphor is an important mode of understanding, structuring and transferring experience is implicitly stated in a comment made by Halliday (1998: 29) about the complex aspects of pain and the sufferer's struggle to unravel them. Thus, for Halliday, pain is not only complex – "it is also very threatening; so we struggle hard to understand it, to assimilate it to other, more domesticated patterns of experience." Though no explicit mention of the term 'metaphor' is made, Halliday's wording basically echoes the cognitive understanding of the function of metaphor as a process whereby a complex conceptual domain is understood in terms of another more recognisable domain of experience. Hence, essentially, there seems to exist a significant degree of correspondence between Halliday's functional perspective and the cognitive linguistic approach with respect to the understanding of conceptual metaphor in structuring experience. This convergence of the two approaches has already been pointed out in relation to various aspects of Halliday's functional account of pain as 'thing' and will become even more apparent as we proceed with the examination and interpretation of the metaphorical linguistic expressions observed in the Greek data.

Given the function of (conceptual and linguistic) metaphor and the widely accepted view that "metaphor is essential for how people communicate about abstract, difficult-to-talk-about ideas and about aspects of ordinary experience" (Gibbs, 1999: 44), it should not come as a surprise that patients have often been observed to use metaphorical language in order to describe their private painful sensation explicitly. This observation has been cited in studies conducted from the perspective of medical sciences (e.g. Borsook, LeBel and McPeek, 1998; Fernandez and Towery, 1996; Melzack and Torgerson, 1971), caring sciences (e.g. Hallberg and Carlsson, 2000; Paulson, Danielson and Söderberg, 2002; Söderberg and Norberg, 1995), and social sciences (e.g. Aldrich and Eccleston, 2000; Kugelmann, 1999). On the basis of what the patients themselves often admit, wherever reported, metaphorical pain language is consistently related to the difficulty of communicating the pain experience, i.e. producing a description by means of which the listener can 'recognise' this private sensation which he cannot access.

Hence, Fernandez and Towery (1996) suggest that "because pain is often so difficult to describe, patients may resort to metaphors in an effort to communicate their experience." Along the same lines, Söderberg and Norberg (1995) interpret the use of metaphorical expressions by fibromyalgia patients as an indication that they have problems expressing their experiences, which is reconfirmed in other studies in the language used by fibromyalgia patients, e.g. Hallberg and Carlsson (2000) and Paulson, Danielson and Söderberg (2002). The descriptions of pain provided by female patients are characterised as often being 'dramatic' in Hallberg and Carlsson (*ibid.*: 32, 35). This dramatic aspect is equally attributed to difficulties in finding words to describe emotions but it is further understood as potentially reflecting "the women's excessive appraisals of the threatening and stressful situation of being in pain." (See also Smith, 1992 and Watson, 1987, for insightful accounts of the power of metaphor in nursing.)

On the other hand, from a social sciences perspective, in his hermeneutical-phenomenological study of the narratives of pain produced by working class people, Kugelmann (1999) reveals how they experience and describe pain, in terms of specific polarities and themes. Though it is not metaphorical language *per se* which is examined but, rather, the way pain is conceived, some of the themes that emerged are metaphorically structured and, hence, highlight my analysis of the metaphorical pain descriptions observed in the Greek data. Similarly, in Aldrich and Eccleston (2000), a social constructionist analysis of how sense is made of everyday pain, eight factors or accounts of pain were derived, some of which will allow us to gain insights into the way pain is conceived in the pain utterances.

It is also noteworthy that, besides pain, illness – and in particular chronic illness – has also been observed to be talked about metaphorically (Sontag, 1978 and 1988, published together in one volume, 1991; Gwyn, 1999): it is the same difficulty of putting intense private human experiences into literal words that has been suggested to motivate the use of metaphorical language as a resource in understanding illness and communicating it to others (Deignan, 2005b: 133). Interestingly, some source domains, e.g. INVASION, EXTERNAL ENEMY, FIRE, MOVEMENT, appear to be applied for the metaphorical representation of both pain and illness (Gwyn, 1999; Sontag, 1991; Semino, Heywood and Short, 2004). (See relevant discussion below.)

To form a clearer image of the metaphorical representations of pain emerging from the various studies referred to above, let us briefly consider some of the most striking and interrelated recurring metaphors. Most of them are also observed in the Greek data, as my subsequent analysis will show.

In particular, for Fabrega and Tyma (1976b), pain is likened to DEFORMATION, DESTRUCTION, DAMAGE, and HARM.[1] Söderberg and Norberg (1995) claim that a similar underlying model where pain entails AGGRESSIVE PHYSICAL DEFORMATION is derived from their Swedish data, adding that VICTIMISATION OF THE PATIENT is a further metaphorical theme related to the pain experience. That individuals communicate their experience of pain as 'damage to their body' is also reported by DeSouza and Frank (2000: 215). In Aldrich and Eccleston (2000), the conceptualisation of PAIN AS DAMAGE and AGGRESSION takes the form of MALFUNCTION, ABUSE, ALIEN INVASION, and, ultimately, leads to the understanding of PAIN AS A STRONG, MALIGN, EXTERNAL, AGENTIC POWER. This metaphorical understanding of pain actually echoes Kern's (1987) idea of PAIN AS AN ATTACK UPON THE BODY AND PERSON, resulting in the personification of PAIN AS A MALEVOLENT AGGRESSOR. Of the metaphorical conceptualisations of pain put forward by Kugelmann (1999), those most frequently recurring in my data are (related to) PAIN AS PRIVATE POSSESSION, INDIGENCE, LOSS, A WAY OF (NOT) DWELLING, CONFINEMENT, i.e. PRISON, and HOMELESSNESS. Finally, the metaphorical representation of PAIN AS A MOVING OBJECT is attested in Söderberg and Norberg (1995: 57). These conceptualisations of pain will be referred to in more detail in my analysis wherever they are borne out by the Greek data.

The observation made in such variously oriented studies that metaphors are extensively used in pain language motivated my preliminary search for metaphorical configurations of pain in the Greek doctor-patient data of my initial sub-corpus, which were in fact found to be abundant in *ponos* 'pain' metaphorical constructions. My subsequent exploration of the extensive corpus on which the present study is based revealed that metaphorical representations of pain were equally very frequent in this material. Having become familiarised with the basic aspects of the metaphorical structuring of pain in the original subset of my Greek data (Lascaratou and Marmaridou, 2005), I was motivated to proceed with a large-scale investigation of the metaphors collected in the new material of my corpus so as to test the validity of earlier claims with additional and more diverse data and within a more elaborate theoretical framework.

In investigating the metaphorical conceptualisation of pain, I am consciously and deliberately using a so-called 'bottom-up' approach. In other words, following the direction of investigation in corpus linguistics, i.e. from form to meaning, I will attempt to trace underlying conceptual metaphors or metaphorical systems through a detailed examination of the *ponos*-related linguistic patterns observed in my cor-

1. It could be argued that such metaphorical representations of pain as DEFORMATION, DESTRUCTION, or DAMAGE are based on the metonymic relation CAUSE FOR EFFECT, given that (tissue) damage / destruction and bodily deformation are the basic causes of pain.

pus of natural language data. This data analysis was based on first reading the corpus end-to-end so as to trace potential clues to patterns and then using them as starting points for automated searches in the electronic corpus by means of concordancing. (See Cameron and Deignan, 2003.) In following this procedure, I am aware that, as Deignan (1999a: 180) remarks, concordancing is "a powerful observational tool, but no more than a tool; a researcher is needed to decide what to examine and how to interpret the resulting data" and that "the corpus linguist needs to be adept in working out how to interrogate the corpus and what to search for" (Deignan, 2005b: 88). (For the contribution of corpus linguistics to the study of metaphor, see Cameron and Deignan, 2003; Deignan, 1999a; 1999b; 2005a; 2005b.)

As was pointed out in Chapter 3, it is the diversity, complexity and multi-faceted nature of pain that makes it necessary to examine the specific constructions naturally produced by a considerable number of ordinary, pain suffering, individuals – either at the time they experience the sensation or when they attempt to describe it – if one wishes to gain a thorough understanding of how this domain of human experience is conceptualised. Despite the apparent shortcomings of such an approach – i.e. that the occurrence of all related significant structures is not ensured, although the procedure is time-consuming and cumbersome – my decision to follow this method of data collection was motivated by the very nature of the universal, yet very private, experience of pain. In other words, it is my belief that looking at the precise linguistic structures employed by *different ordinary* people when they *spontaneously* talk about their pain should be the first step towards comprehending the metaphorical structure of pain language. This does not mean, however, that I suggest that other sources of evidence, such as the ones used in a 'top-down' approach, should be excluded. Far from adopting such a stance, as will be shown below, I will attempt to 'merge' my approach with the 'top-down' one followed by Kövecses (2000) in his analysis of metaphor in emotion, by re-interpreting my findings in the light of the generalisations and cognitive structures suggested in his conclusions.

In a 'top-down' approach, researchers mainly rely on selective evidence provided by highly conventionalised (i.e. not simply conventional) metaphorical linguistic expressions to be found in relevant dictionaries, specially developed corpora, or other lists. Linguistic expressions are referred to as conventionalised, worn-out, or even clichéd metaphors when they are commonly and naturally used by native speakers of a language in everyday life to talk about particular concepts (e.g. life, death, friendship, love, various emotions, etc.). Such linguistic metaphors illustrate the conventional metaphorical conceptualisation of the related concepts by the speakers of a language. Hence, for cognitive scholars, whose main goal is to propose underlying global cognitive structures that may interpret the linguistic data, conventionalised metaphorical expressions constitute a valuable source of evidence for the working of our conceptual system.

Pointing out the limitations of both approaches, namely, that top-down researchers do not see the trees for the wood while bottom-up researchers do not see the wood for the trees, Kövecses (forth.) sees it as a challenge that linguists should combine the two approaches. In particular, he concludes, "it is clear that a top-down approach needs to be supplemented by a bottom-up approach (including, e.g. corpus linguistic studies) for a fuller, more detailed and more precise characterisation of prototypes of happiness and pain, and very likely, for that of many other concepts."

Having already made a beginning along these lines in Lascaratou and Marmaridou (2005) and Lascaratou (forth.), in this chapter I intend to proceed as follows: (a) I will systematically look at the collected *ponos* nominal constructions and derive the specific-level pain metaphors by focusing on the constraints emerging from the grammatical function assigned to *ponos* in various structures; (b) on the basis of Talmy's force dynamic schema (1988) and in the light of Kövecses's (2000) analysis of metaphor in emotion and its application to the investigation of the conceptual structure of pain (Kövecses, forth.), I will attempt to show that the collected Greek pain data provide evidence in support of the view that specific-level pain metaphors are instantiations of such a general metaphor as PAIN IS A FORCE; (c) I will extend to pain the specific and limited sense of 'embodiment' proposed by Kövecses (2000) for emotions, namely, that the conceptualisations of emotions can only emerge *within the constraints* imposed by universal physiology, i.e. that they cannot contradict the functioning of the body in emotions;[2] hence, I will argue that, given the physical aspect of pain – the (actual or potential) tissue damage associated with the painful experience – the specific-level Greek pain metaphors are motivated, i.e. they are constrained, by universal aspects of human physiology

2. See Gibbs (2006) for a systematic exploration of how people's subjective, felt experiences of their bodies in action provide part of the fundamental grounding for human cognition and language. Abundant empirical evidence emerging from a wide range of disciplines (e.g. work on perception, imagery and reasoning, language and communication, emotions and consciousness, and cognitive development) is described in support of the claim that the mind is embodied.

associated with the experience of pain;[3] and, (d) without actually treating discourse-pragmatic factors, it will simply be suggested that the metaphorical construal of pain in doctor-patient interaction appears also to be both discoursally motivated and fully exploited by the interlocutors, the ultimate goal of such interaction being to take control of the threateningly intrusive pain.[4]

Finally, extending Foolen's (1997) account of the externalisation of emotion to the communication of pain by adopting the distinction he draws between the direct, non-verbal mode and the indirect (*via* cognition) verbal channel, I shall assume that in *ponos* constructions the conceptualisation of pain precedes its verbalisation, i.e. that such configurations constitute a cognitively motivated indirect channel of externalising pain. Hence, I shall argue that it is the conceptualisation of pain, rather than the painful experience itself, which is communicated when pain is externalised by means of explicit, objectifying descriptions, in particular metaphorically motivated *ponos* constructions. On the basis of additional linguistic, cognitive and discursive evidence, I shall support the identification of *ponos* metaphorical structures with the extreme pole representing the descriptive function in the proposed integrating continuum of pain manifestations, the other pole featuring automatic reactions such as the primitive cry.

8.2 The conceptual grounding of *ponos* metaphors and their linguistic realisation

In this section I shall examine the metaphorical understanding of pain as it emerges from the analysis of *ponos* 'pain' nominal constructions used by the interlocutors in my Greek corpus of doctor-patient dialogues. This account is restricted to pat-

3. As was mentioned in Chapter 3 (footnote 4), one cannot rule out the possibility that the focus on musculoskeletal pain data – not originally intended but rather a consequence of some physicians' refusal to participate in the project and the data collection – may have constrained the observed linguistic manifestations of pain to some unknown extent. Hence, though challenging, it is beyond the scope of this study to compare systematically the sets of metaphors used to talk about different types of pain and potentially propose – if that is the case – different conceptual construals (and possibly the corresponding lexico-grammatical forms) as predominantly underlying the linguistic metaphors used to describe pains related to different organs or different systems of the human body, e.g. earaches, toothaches, headaches, sciatica or other forms of neuralgia.

4. In a clearly discourse-oriented analysis of pain related doctor-patient interaction, it would be useful to consider more specific, lower-level, discourse goals (e.g. describing a pain in response to a question posed by the doctor, trying to get the medical expert to stop doing something which is causing pain at that moment, trying to get the health professional prescribe the appropriate pain relief treatment) and examine if these could serve to distinguish between different types of linguistic structure.

terns containing the noun *ponos*, with a view to examining a specific aspect of the relation between conceptual and linguistic pain metaphors, namely, the role played by the grammatical function assigned to *ponos* in different structures. Hence, the focus will be on how the various conceptualisations of the experience are constrained by the grammaticalisation of *ponos* as object or subject in the relevant transitive / intransitive constructions observed in the material of this study.[5]

With additional data collected from the dialogues of the new material, it will be possible to confirm that *ponos* nominal constructions are systematically motivated by both language-specific syntactico-semantic constraints and conceptual metaphors. The evidence derived from the whole corpus of the present study will reinforce the claim that the construal of pain as a thing realised through the noun *ponos* 'pain' lends itself to the objectification of pain and leads to its conceptualisation mostly as A HIGHLY DISTINGUISHABLE UNDESIRABLE POSSESSED ENTITY and as AN EXTERNAL-TO-THE-SELF MOVING FORCE capable of INVADING the individual as AN UNINVITED INTRUDER, ultimately acting as A MALEVOLENT AGGRESSOR, A TORTURER, and AN IMPRISONING ENEMY.

The fact that this analysis focuses on metaphorical correlates of the nominal construal of pain should not be misinterpreted as suggesting that it is assumed that the metaphorical correlates of the verbal construal of pain are not likewise revealing about how pain is conceptualised. My interest in focusing on *ponos* nominal constructions stems from their significance in doctor-patient discourse as observed in the Greek corpus: the objectification of *ponos* through the ontological metaphor motivates the representation of pain as an entity identifiable in terms of certain properties, i.e. in concrete and 'objective' terms. Thus, it will be claimed, the importance of the construal of pain as an objectified entity rather than a holistic experience – and perhaps its most significant justification – in doctor-patient interaction is that it facilitates the interlocutors in their attempt to identify, describe, or define the private sensation of pain, i.e. to treat it in concrete and socially shared terms.

8.2.1 The grammaticalisation of *ponos* as object of the verbs *exo*, *esθanome*, and *njoθo*

Let us now proceed with the examination of constructions where *ponos* is the syntactic object of such transitive verbs as *esθanome*, *njoθo*, and *exo*. (For an initial

5. This particular focus on *ponos* nominal constructions was originally motivated by the observation (mentioned at the end of Chapter 7) that, in the naturally-occurring data of the corpus, *ponos* is configured as the Actor in processes of 'doing' or 'doing something to some other entity' only in metaphorically structured utterances.

account of these constructions, see Lascaratou and Marmaridou, 2005.) The conceptual grounding of these constructions where pain is objectified will pave the way for the metaphorical understanding of pain as an agentive power, separate from the sufferer's self and, ultimately, its personification. Consider:

(1) P: *esθanθika* enan aforito *pono* eδo.
feel-PST:1SG an unbearable pain-ACC here
'*I felt* an unbearable *pain* here.'

(2) D: *njoθis* eki *pono*?
feel-PRS:2SG there pain-ACC
'*Do you feel pain* there?'

(3) P: δen ton *ixa afton ton pono.*
not it-ACC have-PST:1SG this the pain-ACC
'*I* didn't *have this pain.*'

In the light of Haiman's (1983) principle of iconicity, constructions featuring *ponos* as direct object of the verbs *esθanome* and *njoθo* can be seen as a first step towards introducing a conceptual distance between the sufferer's self and his pain sensation. They are a linguistic means whereby the sufferer's self and his pain, realised by separate constituents, are iconically represented as two separate entities. Thus, clauses containing these verbs which denote the experiencing of a sensation, e.g. (1) and (2), are, in functional terms, mental processes of perception profiling pain as that which is sensed – the Phenomenon – in the form of the grammatical object, whereas the sufferer's self is the Senser, grammaticalised as the verb suffix.

The iconic distancing between the Senser and his experience expressed in such constructions is brought out more vividly if we compare them to *ponao* utterances in any of their two basic functional interpretations: in the relational: attributive understanding, the *ponao* bare verb form realises simultaneously three elements, namely, the Process itself, the sufferer's self as the Carrier of pain construed as Attribute, and the Attribute conflated with the Process. On the other hand, in the material process interpretation, pain is structured as a self-engendering Process carried out by the sufferer from within. Hence, the linguistic realisation of the sufferer's self and his sensation as one lexemic unit in *ponao* constructions iconically reflects the sufferer's involvement in the painful experience, which is not the case in *esθanome* / *njoθo* + *ponos* constructions, e.g. (4).[6] Compare the occurrence of both patterns in example (5):

6. This difference is essentially related to the syntactico-semantic properties of *ponao* vs. those of *esθanome* / *njoθo*, the former being a prototypically intransitive verb, while the latter are transitive ones, requiring a complement.

(4) P: *esθanome pono* mesa.
feel-PRS:1SG pain-ACC inside
'*I feel pain* inside.'

(5) D: e, *ponesate*? *njosate pono*?
hmm hurt-PST:2PL feel-PST:2PL pain-ACC
'Hmm, *did you hurt* (*did that hurt you*)? *Did you feel any pain*?'

However, due to the semantic affinity between the verbs *esθanome* / *njoθo*, as verbs of 'sensing', and *ponos*, as a noun denoting a sensation, the distance between the sufferer's self and his pain is not as prominently profiled as it is in the case of *exo* + *ponos* constructions. As we shall see below, this difference is further reinforced by the fine distinction between the semantic shades expressed by *ponos* when it co-occurs with *esθanome* / *njoθo* as compared to when it co-occurs with *exo*.

Though *exo* + *ponos* patterns were analysed in Chapter 7 within the functional paradigm as relational: attributive processes of the possessive type, a more thorough analysis of their semantic features will shed light on the subtle nuances involved. Thus, we shall be able to trace the emergence of an understanding of pain as an alienable possession leading to its objectification, which in turn will motivate its construal as an entity identifiable in terms of certain properties, finally acquiring the ability to take action.

The semantic construals of the *exo* + *ponos* construction as a whole depend on the syntactico-semantic features of its parts, i.e. *exo* and *ponos*, which appear to be closely associated as two interrelated determining factors. In particular, *ponos* may be construed as profiling the sensation either as a type of feeling or as a particular instance (or instances) of a feeling (Langacker, 1991). In the case of Greek nouns, when it is type of feeling that needs to be specified, this is typically expressed in the bare singular form of the noun, whereas instantiation of feeling is grammatically realised by means of pluralisation and the use of (definite or indefinite) determiners and modifiers (see Marmaridou, 1984).

It is worth noting here a significant difference between *exo* + *ponos* and *esθanome* / *njoθo* + *ponos* constructions, which in fact reinforces the understanding of the former as a configuration whereby pain is more distinctly objectified. To be more specific, while with *esθanome* / *njoθo* the pain sensation is often construed as a type, rather than an instance, of feeling – by virtue of the co-occurring bare form of *ponos*, e.g. (6) – this is rarely the case with *exo*, which clearly favours the understanding of *ponos* as a particular instance of the experience, e.g. (7) where *ponos* is pluralised. Notably, it appears that the infrequent co-occurrence of *exo* with the bare form of *ponos* is preferred in negative patterns, such as (8). Consider:

(6) D: *ti njoθis?*
what feel-PRS:2SG
'*What do you feel?*'

P: *pono, pono.*
pain-ACC pain-ACC
'*Pain, pain.*'

(7) P: eno sto xorio... *ixa δinatus ponus* ke ti nixta akomi.
whereas at-the village-ACC have-PST:1SG strong pains-ACC and the night-ACC even
'Whereas at my village... even at night *I had strong pains.*'

(8) D: na mu pite, mexri pote isaste kala ke *δen ixate pono?*
to-PARTCL I-GEN say-PFV:NON-PST:2PL until when be-PST:2PL well and not have-PST:2PL pain-ACC
'Tell me, until when were you well without *having (any) pain?*'

As for *exo*, it may also be semantically construed in two ways: it may be interpreted either as a semantically empty linking verb, i.e. one characterised by loss of lexical meaning (see Moser, 1993 and Theophanopoulou-Kontou, 1988), or as primarily possessive (see Nikiforidou, 1991 and Veloudis, 2003). Though both semantic construals of *exo* were observed in the data, it is the possessive one which is of central importance in the analysis of the metaphorical understanding of *ponos*. Thus, in the majority of *exo + ponos* constructions, *exo* is interpreted as possessive, this semantic analysis being motivated by *ponos* nominals profiling pain as a particular instantiation of a feeling. On the other hand, the grammaticalisation of pain as type of feeling in the bare form of *ponos* nominals motivates the relational understanding of *exo*.

Moving on to a further semantic feature of *ponos*, namely, its understanding as an alienable or inalienable entity, it is plausible to assume that the former is associated with the possessive construal of *exo* and the latter with its relational semantics (see Brugman, 1988). If all the interrelated and interdependent semantic aspects of *ponos* and *exo* discussed above are combined, it emerges that *exo + ponos* constructions are predominantly configured as possessive processes of a particular type: in these the sufferer's self – grammaticalised as subject in the verb suffix – is profiled as the possessor of an alienable rather than inalienable possession – grammaticalised as syntactic object. The patient's ultimate goal being to bring pain under his control (Brugman, *ibid.*), it seems plausible to interpret such possessive constructions as linguistic devices whereby the objectified painful experience is configured as being positioned within the possessor's sphere of influence (Langacker, 1975). Hence, the metaphor PAIN IS A POSSESSION / A POSSESSED OBJECT is instantiated.

At this point, it seems natural to associate the application of the source domain POSSESSION OF AN OBJECT to the conceptualisation of the existence of pain (e.g. *I have a terrible pain*) with the application of the same domain to express the 'existence' of an emotion (e.g. *He has a lot of trouble / anxieties*). According to Kövecses (2000: 36, 41) the metaphor EXISTENCE OF EMOTION IS POSSESSION OF AN OBJECT / POSSESSING AN OBJECT is one of the three major and very general metaphors that have as their main focus the existence of emotion and apply to all emotion concepts, the other two being EXISTENCE OF EMOTION IS PRESENCE HERE and EXISTENCE OF EMOTION IS BEING IN A BOUNDED SPACE, which we shall deal with later on in our discussion. These source domains are not unique to emotion concepts; they are part of the way we conceptualise events in general (i.e. states, changes of states, actions, etc.) as put forth by Lakoff (1990, 1993) in the EVENT STRUCTURE metaphor in English. Therefore, emotions being conceptualised as states (i.e. emotional states), *inter alia*, it is plausible that these very general metaphors should also apply to emotions.

To capture the various aspects of the metaphor EXISTENCE OF EMOTION IS POSSESSION OF AN OBJECT / A POSSESSED OBJECT let us trace its emergence within the EVENT STRUCTURE metaphor. Thus, a state, e.g. an emotional, physical, social, etc. state, can be viewed as an attribute, i.e. as an attributed state. This understanding of states as attributes motivates their conceptualisation as objects that may be given, acquired, owned, possessed, preserved, and lost. Hence, the metaphor ATTRIBUTES ARE POSSESSED OBJECTS. Given the conceptualisation of emotions as states, the metaphor (EXISTENCE OF) EMOTION IS A POSSESSED OBJECT emerges as an instantiation of the higher-level metaphor ATTRIBUTES ARE POSSESSED OBJECTS. Pain being defined as an experience with an emotional aspect, it is natural that, like other emotions, it should also be understood as an attributed state and, therefore, as A POSSESSED OBJECT.

That pain is understood as a possession has also been argued by Halliday (1998) within his functional analysis of pain as thing, as we saw in Chapter 7. It is worth pointing out that this representation of pain is suggested by Halliday not only in his discussion of the proposed seven grammatically construed semantic properties of pain, but also in his interpretation of the structural configurations featuring 'pain' as participant. In particular, the concepts of 'attribution' and 'possession' are invoked to identify such expressions as *I've got a headache* and *that gives me a headache* as relational: attributive / possessive processes and relational: attributive / possessive / agentive processes, respectively.

To return to our *exo* + *ponos* constructions, once *ponos*, as the grammatical object of the possessive *exo*, is construed as a possessed entity separate from the sufferer's self, it gains distance from him, becoming a referent in discourse independent of the sufferer's self. As an object in the patient's possession, it may be talked about, e.g. (9). What is more, being conceived as an object, it is characterised by a number of properties / features in terms of which it may be described, e.g. (10), or even measured, e.g. (11). These features (cf. Halliday's grammatically construed semantic properties of pain, e.g. its construal as either a bounded or an unbounded thing, as a possession, and as an entity having variable qualities) appear to be directly motivated by the ontological metaphor, not only conceptually and linguistically but also discoursally:

(9) P: mi *mu ksanamilisis j'afton ton pono*!
not I-GEN talk-again-IMP:2SG for this the pain-ACC
'Don't *talk to me about this pain again*!'

(10) D: *kane mu mja periγrafi tu ponu.*
make-IMP:2SG I-GEN a description-ACC the pain-GEN
'*Make (for) me a description of the pain*.'

(11) D: *ti vaθmo θa tu valume tu ponu* apo 0 mexri 10?
what score-ACC shall it-GEN assign-PRS:1PL the pain-GEN from 0 to 10
'*What score shall we assign to the pain* from 0 to 10?'

Hence, with respect to doctor-patient interaction, the importance of the objectification of *ponos* through its understanding as A (POSSESSED) OBJECT is that it enables the interlocutors to treat the subjective sensation of pain in socially shared terms (see also Lascaratou and Marmaridou, 2005). Construed as an objectified entity rather than a holistic experience, pain lends itself to being described, defined or identified in concrete and publicly accepted terms, so as to be controlled and, ultimately, eliminated.

Finally, the possessive understanding of pain is put forth by researchers approaching the issue from different, non-linguistic, perspectives. For example, in Kugelmann's (1999: 1669, 1674) hermeneutical-phenomenological study of pain, it is claimed that pain is experienced by individuals primarily as their private property, "with little cash value", however. Moreover, not only does the individual not become 'richer' by means of this property, but he must also somehow prove its existence in an objective manner if it is to be treated as a social reality. In other words, if the sufferer wishes to be heard and receive proper treatment as a form of justice in response to his complaints, he must strive hard to produce objective evidence that, despite its invisibility, pain exists.

Interestingly, in Paulson, Danielson and Soderberg (2002: 245–246) we come across the concept of possession in relation to illness, viewed from a different, yet, I believe, closely related angle:

> In health, the presence of the lived body is characterised paradoxically by its absence – a healthy body is taken for granted (Leder, 1990). In illness, the relation to the body is changed: Rather than *being* one's body, men are confronted with *hav-*

> *ing* a body in a different way than when healthy. It means losing the familiar "feeling of myself" and expressing a sense of discontinuity with the world.

Thus, it appears that, while in health the individual identifies himself with his body in the sense that body and self are inseparable, in illness the patient becomes conscious of the existence of his body (or certain parts of it) as a possession confronting him from a distance. If we associate this understanding of 'having a body' in illness with 'having pain', we may suggest that the patient conceptualises the existence of either his body or his pain in terms of an unpleasant possession constantly reminding him that he is the unfortunate owner.

This possessive construal of pain and of the body in illness is manifestly illustrated in the following extract from a doctor-patient dialogue:

(12) D: *exete* ala *provlimata ijias*, kiria…?
have-PRS:2PL other problems-ACC health-GEN Mrs
'*Have you got any other health problems*, Mrs…?'
P: oxi. *ixa* arketa xronia prin *ti sponδliki mu stili.*
no have-PST:1SG some years-ACC before the spine-ACC my
'No. Some years ago *I had* (*I suffered from*) *my spine*.'
D: malista.
all right
'All right.'
P: *ixa sponδiloarθritiδa.*
have-PST:1SG ankylosing spondylitis
'*I had ankylosing spondylitis*.'
D: malista. *exete karδia, exete ipertasi, exete kati…?*
all right have-PRS:2PL heart-ACC have-PRS:2PL high-blood-pressure-ACC have-PRS:2PL something- ACC
'All right. *Do you have heart* (*problems*), *do you have high blood pressure, do you have anything else…?*'
P: e, oxi, *ipertasi δen exo.*
hmm no high-blood-pressure-ACC not have-PRS:1SG
'Hmm, no, *I don't have high blood pressure*.'

As we can see, potential or actual health problems (ankylosing spondylitis and high blood pressure) and potentially or actually suffering parts or organs of the patient's body (her spine and her heart) are equally construed as possessions through identical structural configurations.

8.2.2 The grammaticalisation of *ponos* as subject in intransitive structures

That pain, as an objectified entity, gains further distance and independence from the sufferer's self is simultaneously reflected in and motivated by structures where it is grammatically realised as the subject of intransitive verbs. So far, as grammatical object in *esθanome, njoθo, exo, periγrafo, vaθmoloγo, metro*, etc. transitive patterns, *ponos* was configured as the entity to which the patient's action was extended (Goal), or as the patient's possessed Attribute, or as the Phenomenon being sensed. As subject of intransitive structures, *ponos* is now 'promoted' to the initiator or doer (Actor) of processes, that is, of actions. As actions form part of (i.e. are components or aspects of) the EVENT STRUCTURE metaphor in that they are intentionally produced events, the metaphor PAIN IS AN EVENT is activated. Examples (13)-(16) distinctly indicate that pain is conceptualised as an event bounded in time, with a clear beginning and ending, i.e. one that may be identified in terms of its temporal location.

(13) D: ke pote *ksekinise o ponos*?
and when start-PST:3SG the pain-NOM
'And when *did the pain start*?'

(14) D: *sinexizi o ponos* ametavlitos mera nixta?
continue-PRS:3SG the pain-NOM unchanged-NOM day night-ACC
'*Does the pain continue* day and night unchanged?'

(15) P: e, meta *stamatise o ponos*, ala meta apo liγa xronia *ksana* liγo liγo…
hmm afterwards stop-PST:3SG the pain-NOM but after few years-ACC again little little
'Hmm, *the pain stopped* later, but a few years after, *again* gradually…'

(16) P: mu ixe *perasi o ponos* ke meta mu *ksanarxise* pali.
I-GEN have-PST:3SG pass-PFV the pain-NOM and afterwards I-GEN restart-PST:3SG again
'*The pain had passed* (*had left me*) and then *it started again*.'

Furthermore, like emotions, pain manifests variable intensity, which belongs to the extremely general dimensions or aspects of experience in general, and emotions in particular, along with existence, control, passivity, difficulty, harm, etc. (see Kövecses, 2000: 41–2, 193). In the Greek doctor-patient data it is observed that people use a number of different source domains to describe pain intensity and its increase / decrease. Hence various conceptualisations of *ponos* which lend themselves to highlighting intensity are activated. Thus, as our examples illustrate, *ponos* may be perceived as a fluctuating SUBSTANCE, i.e. typically *increasing* and *decreasing* in AMOUNT / QUANTITY (17), A LIVING ORGANISM capable of *growing*

(18), or a NATURAL / PHYSICAL FORCE with variable intensity which is perceived as STRENGTH OF EFFECT (19):

(17) D: *o ponos afksani?*
the pain-NOM increase-PRS:3SG
'*Does the pain increase?*'

(18) P: otan kaθiso *aftos o iδjos o ponos meyaloni…*
when sit-down-PFV:NON-PST:1SG this the same the pain-NOM grow-PRS:3SG
'Whenever I sit down, *this very pain grows bigger…*'

(19) P: *i poni* arxisan na *δinamonun.*
the pains-NOM start-PST:3PL to-PARTCL get-stronger-PRS:3PL
'*The pains* started to *get stronger.*'

The concept HEAT being one of the source domains that focus on the intensity aspect of emotional experience in general, it also applies to pain, as observed in the data. In the case of pain, as I will argue in the next section, this metaphorical understanding of pain intensity and/or of pain itself seems to be motivated by the sensory aspect of the experience. In other words, in the light of Kövecses (2000: 164–5, 185, 190–1 and forth.), I will suggest that the body's physiological functioning in pain, i.e. particular types of tissue damage which are the cause of the painful experience and their accompanying sensory effects, may impose constraints on the way pain is metaphorically conceptualised. In that sense, if the tissue damage produces a sensation of heat, the concept HEAT / FIRE may be applied metonymically as the source domain for the metaphorical structuring of the pain experience. In particular, it seems that it is severe pain intensity that motivates the metaphorical structuring of PAIN as HEAT, or even BLAZING FIRE, as illustrated in examples (20), (21), and (22) which are instances of the metaphor PAIN IS HEAT / FIRE, with (22) depicting its burning effect:[7]

7. When used transitively, the primary meaning of the verb *zvino* which appears in examples (20) and (21) is 'to make something stop burning or being burnt,' i.e. 'to extinguish' / 'to put out' a fire or a light, 'to turn / switch off' a light. When used intransitively, as is the case in both examples above, it means 'to stop burning or being burnt,' i.e. 'to be extinguished' / 'to be put out' / 'to become extinct,' 'to be turned / switched off.' Hence, in (20) and (21) the metaphor PAIN IS HEAT / FIRE is activated by virtue of the presence of the verb *zvino*. I am aware, however, that in the English gloss I have used ('to fade away') part of the semantic content of the Greek verb is missing, as the former is chiefly associated with loss of colour, freshness or vigour. With respect to the source domain of HEAT / FIRE, it is also interesting to note that, to interpret examples containing the verb *erupt* in their corpus of conversations about cancer, Semino, Heywood and Short (2004: 1285) assume the existence of two specific-level metaphors, namely, CANCER IS VOLCANO and CANCER IS FIRE deriving from a conventional CANCER IS HOT / BURNING ENTITY superordinate metaphor.

(20) P: *o ponos ezvise*, o alos, o δikos mu.
the pain-NOM get-extinguished-PST:3SG the other-NOM the mine my
'*The pain has faded away*, the other, my own.'

(21) P: ponai staθera eki. xoris na *zvini*.
hurt-PRS:3SG constantly there without to-PARTCL get-extinguished-PRS:3SG
'It hurts there constantly. Without *fading away*.'

(22) P: *kapsimo* exo eδo.
burn-ACC have-PRS:1SG here
'I've got *something burning* here.'

In the case of extremely severe pain intensity, the concept of MADNESS / INSANITY may be invoked to represent the gravity of the painful condition, thus leading to the metaphor BEING IN PAIN IS BEING INSANE, as shown in the following examples. What this metaphor actually depicts is the psychological situation that the patient is driven to as a result of excruciating pain. It is, therefore, the mental effect of severe pain that is represented by this metaphor and, consequently, pain is understood as an entity that is forceful enough to bring about such extreme effects, which essentially motivates an understanding of pain as a FORCE.

(23) P: kseris ti pono! *trela pono*![8]
know-PRS:2SG what pain-ACC madness pain-ACC
'You know what kind of pain! *Pain* (*which is*) *madness!*'

(24) P: ponai xoris na… xoris *trela* δilaδi.
hurt-PRS:3SG without to-PARTCL without madness-ACC that-is
'It hurts without (causing)… without *madness*, that is.'

The association of pain intensity with MADNESS / INSANITY and HEAT / FIRE will recur in our account as a form of torment used by *ponos* when profiled as a TORTURER. Both metaphors, together with most of the other pain metaphors, will be reconsidered below within the force dynamic schema.

Physical space, together with physical movement, and physical force are basic concepts in terms of which events are understood. It is not surprising, therefore, that these three source domains are employed for the metaphorical structuring of pain as well, as will be shown in the course of our analysis.

In particular, physical space plays a very crucial role in the conceptualisation of pain, since by definition pain has a delimited space, i.e. the human body, within which it may 'occur' or 'be located'. Given the basic 'image-schema' derived from

8. For an analysis of this Greek construction as a 'loose appositional compound' having an exclamatory function, see Chapter 7, note 9.

our interactions with the physical world whereby we experience our physical selves (i.e. our bodies and body organs) as containers – hence THE HUMAN BODY IS A CONTAINER and PEOPLE ARE CONTAINERS – it is only natural that we should also conceptualise the sufferer's body as a container, one within the boundaries of which pain occurs or resides. (See also Lascaratou and Marmaridou, 2005.)

The importance of the container image-schema as a source domain for the understanding of human experience becomes apparent from the central role played by the metaphor THE HUMAN BODY IS A CONTAINER in the conceptualisation of emotions in many unrelated languages in the world. The "'inside–outside' perspective for the human body" defined by the container image, Kövecses (2000: 37) argues, emerges as a near-universal way of viewing the body in relation to emotions. Thus, the body is conceptualised as a container inside which emotions exist / occur; hence the widely observed metaphor EMOTION IS A SUBSTANCE IN A CONTAINER. Given that pain is not only physically linked to the body as the bounded space within which it is actually sensed but it also has a fundamental emotional aspect, the near-universal way of conceptualising THE BODY AS A CONTAINER (FOR EMOTIONS) provides further motivation for the understanding of THE (SUFFERER'S) BODY AS A CONTAINER (for pain).

It could be argued, however, that in the case of typical emotions (e.g. anger, joy, etc.), such a conceptualisation of the human body is straightforwardly metaphorical (even though bodily based), while in the case of pain, the expressions related to its location inside the body could hardly be considered metaphorical, as (some) pains can literally be located inside the body. In other words, one might contend that in proposing the container image-schema for the understanding of the locus of pain, the distinction between emotions and physical sensations such as (physical) pain is insufficiently taken into account. Far from disregarding this subtle distinction and the fact that physical pain has a literally physical location, i.e. the human body, I essentially propose here that the container image-schema is instantiated for the understanding of the locus of pain when the ontological metaphor discussed above is applied in its various forms for the representation of pain. What is more, the container image-schema best captures a subtle aspect of the pain sensation which seems to emerge from such metaphorical representations of pain, namely, that pain appears as being 'contained' rather than simply 'located' in the body.

Hence, assuming the various versions of the ontological metaphor, namely, PAIN IS A SUBSTANCE / A LIVING ORGANISM / A FORCE / HEAT / FIRE, and the container image metaphor THE BODY IS A CONTAINER, I propose that the locus of pain may be conceptualised through the metaphor PAIN IS A SUBSTANCE / A FORCE / etc. IN A CONTAINER. It is noteworthy that, from his historical semantic perspective and on the basis of both historical evidence and present-day English data, Peters (2004: 198–199) also suggests that the experience of pain, understood as A QUAN-

TITY – increasing / decreasing and filling the body – is related to the metaphorical representation of THE BODY AS A CONTAINER.

Consider the following examples where the key words *eδo mesa* 'here inside / in here', primarily used to refer to bounded physical spaces, could be seen as evidence of Kövecses's (2000: 37) suggested 'inside–outside' perspective for the human body as defined by the container image:

(25) P: ke o ponos aftos ine *eδo… eδo mesa.*
and the pain this-NOM be-PRS:3SG here here inside
'And this pain is *here… here inside.*'

(26) P: tora *eki epikendrono* ton pono *kapu. eki. eδo. eδo mesa.*
now there locate-PRS:1SG the pain-ACC somewhere there here here inside
'Now *I can pinpoint* the pain (as being) *somewhere there. There. Here. Here inside.*'

(27) P: esθanome ke pali pono *eδo mesa.*
feel-PRS:1SG and again pain-ACC here inside
'I'm feeling pain again *here inside.*'

On the basis of the corpus data, it is suggested, once more, that this conceptualisation of THE SUFFERER'S BODY AS A CONTAINER FOR PAIN may be associated with the lexico-grammatical analysis of the location of pain provided by Halliday (1998), the former offering a cognitive interpretation for the latter. Moreover, the objectification of *ponos* through the ontological metaphor, in general, and the container image-schema it structures, in particular, motivate the representation of pain in 'objective' terms that may effectively be exploited in doctor-patient interaction.

In addition to being the locus of pain, for Aldrich and Eccleston (2002: 1632), "the body is the centre or focus of explanation and representation" as it sets physical and representational boundaries within which the modern self is contained. We will be coming back to this conceptualisation of the body in our subsequent analysis of pain as aggressor or intruder. (See also the discussion of the relation between body and self in relation to pain in section 6.3.)

Moreover, the location of an object in space also entails its motion within it. Hence, the metaphorical representation of the pain experience in terms of motion may be associated with this basic mode of perceiving reality, which is derived from the physical domain of conceptual structure. It emerges from the data under (28)-(32) derived from our doctor-patient dialogues that the metaphor PAIN IS A MOVING ENTITY is instantiated. (See Lascaratou and Marmaridou, 2005 for a first interpretation of the metaphorical representation of pain in terms of motion leading to its personification, further elaborated below.)

In particular, within the EVENT STRUCTURE metaphor, physical MOVEMENT into or out of a bounded space is used as a source domain for the metaphorical representation of the concept of CHANGE. Thus, the submetaphor CHANGES ARE MOVEMENTS applies to changes from one state to another, e.g. from a non-emotional to an emotional state, as in *falling in despair / into disgrace / out of love*. I suggest that physical MOVEMENT is also extended to the experience of pain to conceptualise the change from a pain-free to a painful state. However, unlike emotions, in the case of pain it is not the (sufferer's) self which is understood as moving but rather pain itself. Physical MOVEMENT, therefore, applies to the conceptualisation of the onset and the subsidence of pain on the basis of the two metaphors THE SUFFERER'S BODY IS A CONTAINER (FOR PAIN) and PAIN IS A MOVING ENTITY. Example (28) provides a very vivid image of the onset of pain, its subsidence, and eventual recurrence, in terms of the movement of *ponos* 'into', 'out of', and 'back into' the bounded space of the BODY-CONTAINER:

(28) P: *erxete o ponos, fevji, ksanarxete.*
come-PRS:3SG the pain-NOM go-PRS:3SG come-again-PRS:3SG
'*The pain comes and goes, comes back again.*'

In the case of pain, MOVEMENT is further motivated by its construal as a FORCE having an origin / source and a final destination / goal. Thus, the source – path – goal image schema is activated: PAIN is configured as an entity, a FORCE that *comes* and *goes*; it may *pass through* or *approach* particular positions, *spread* in various directions (e.g. in lower, higher or deeper sites), and finally *end up* in other parts of the suffering body. The following are typical instantiations of the source – path – goal image schema:

(29) P: *plisiazi o ponos* pros ta kato liγo.
come-close-PRS:3SG the pain-NOM toward the down a-bit
'*The pain comes closer* further down a bit.'

(30) P: …etsi *aplonete o ponos* ke meta me xtipai eδo sto xeri.
like-that spread-PRS:3SG the pain-NOM and then I-ACC strike-PRS:3SG here at-the arm-ACC
'…*the pain spreads* like that and then it strikes me here in the arm.'

(31) D: *ftani* mexri ta δaxtila?
reach-PRS:3SG as-far-as the fingers-ACC
'*Does it reach* as far as the fingers?'

(32) P: mu *pai pjo vaθia o ponos…*
I-GEN go-PRS:3SG more deep the pain-NOM
'*The pain goes deeper* (inside me)…'

It is worth noting that very similar representations of PAIN AS A MOVING ENTITY are also reported in Söderberg and Norberg (1995: 57): "The pain was related as being spread all over the body or as wandering from one location to another." Similarly, the source domain of MOVEMENT (IN SPACE) is also used to talk about the spread of cancer, as observed in the analysis of metaphors in a corpus of conversations about this terminal disease (Semino, Heywood and Short, 2004: 1277–1280). However, Semino, Heywood and Short argue that the boundary between literal and metaphorical language is very fuzzy in relation to the development of cancer, as it often involves the literal movement of cells inside the body. (See also Sontag, 1991: 15, for an understanding of the principal cancer metaphors as referring to topography: "cancer 'spreads' or 'proliferates' or is 'diffused' [...].")[9] It might be argued that, likewise, in the case of pain there is nothing metaphorical about saying that a pain 'moves' or 'spreads (out)'. Yet, even if one accepts some degree of fuzziness in the boundary between the literal and metaphorical understanding of such pain expressions, it seems to me that the situation is quite different here: there is no literal movement of pain stimuli inside the body but rather the sensation may be felt in various parts of the body. The existence of simultaneously or consecutively aching points in the body leads to the delineation of a path or multiple paths along which pain, as if it were a distinct moving entity, is ultimately conceptualised as 'passing through' or 'travelling'.

Depending on the lexico-grammatical features of a proposition, MOVEMENT may be represented either as self-propelled, i.e. caused by the moving entity itself, or as resulting from the action of some external entity or force, i.e. as other-propelled. (For an analysis of Greek motion verbs, see Antonopoulou, 1987.) By virtue of its function as grammatical subject of motion verbs in the processes presented above, *ponos* is profiled as the initiator of motion, as the doer of the actions, i.e. as the Actor, in functional terms. Similarly, within the EVENT STRUCTURE metaphor, self-propelled movement is used as a source domain for the metaphorical conceptualisation of actions, that is, of intentionally produced events.

It is precisely its grammaticalisation as subject and, hence, its construal as initiator of its own movement that allows PAIN to be further configured not simply as A MOVING OBJECT, but most importantly as A VOLUNTARY, SELF-WILLED and, therefore, ANIMATE ENTITY. Consequently, the ontological metaphor of personification, PAIN IS AN ANIMATE AGENT, is activated.

Personification of pain derived from its metaphorical representation as A MOVING ENTITY is also assumed by Fabrega and Tyma (1976b: 366, 368) for the

9. According to Sontag (1991: 15), cancer is not so much represented metaphorically as a disease of time but rather "as a disease or pathology of space."

analysis of such intransitive motion patterns as *the / a pain ran / raced / jumped / leapt through my arm / leg / stomach / body etc.*:

> ...the experience has been anthropomorphosized to the point that the experience can be conceived of as an agent capable of "performing" an action. The implication here is that the experience of pain is active, energized and dynamic.

Since pain shows up in the sufferer's body typically without any previous notice or invitation, and randomly moves around, unexpectedly settling in various locations where it is unwanted, it is further metaphorically understood as AN INTRUDER, AN UNDESIRED, UNINVITED AND UNWELCOME VISITOR, who *appears* and *disappears arbitrarily*, actually invading the sufferer's self. Consider the following:

(33) P: *aftos o ponos erxete apotoma...* pote *erxete* pote *fevji*.
this the pain-NOM come-PRS:3SG suddenly sometimes come-PRS:3SG sometimes go-away-PRS:3SG
'*This pain comes suddenly...* sometimes *it comes*, sometimes *it goes away*.'

(34) P: *perna enas ponos...* ke me sfazi.
pass-PRS:3SG a pain-NOM and I-ACC slaughter-PRS:3SG
'*A pain passes...* and slaughters me.'

(35) P: ine tria xronia peripu pu *mu parusiastikane poni*.
be-PRS:3PL three years-NOM about that I-GEN appear-PST:3PL pains-NOM
'It's been almost three years since *pains appeared to me*.'

(36) P: *δen exi eksafanisti aftos o ponos*.
not have-PRS:3SG disappear-PFV this the pain-NOM
'*This pain has not disappeared*.'

The following extract vividly shows the sufferer's apprehension that pain may unexpectedly recur and the resulting feeling of isolation he experiences (*eyo zo ston kozmo mu* 'I live in a world of my own'):

(37) P: afu kamja fora kaθomaste sto spiti ke vlepume tileorasi ke *eyo zo ston kozmo mu* ke sizitao ke leo "oreos o ponos aftos, axu na mu *erxotane alos enas* etsi ke *na 'fevje*." meta apo liγo *ksanarxete pali o iδjos*.
since some time-ACC sit-PRS:1PL in-the house-ACC and watch-PRS:1PL television-ACC and I-NOM live-PRS:1SG in-the world-ACC my and discuss-PRS:1SG and say-PRS:1SG nice-NOM the pain this-NOM wish to-PARTCL I-GEN come-IPFV:3SG other one-NOM like-this and to-PARTCL go-IPFV:3SG after from little come-back-PRS:3SG again the same-NOM
'Imagine, sometimes, while we are sitting at home watching television, *I live in a world of my own* (am alone with my thoughts) and I say to myself

> "what a nice pain this is, I wish if *another one came* that *it would go* like this." After a while, *the same old one comes back*.'

As we shall see in the remaining part of the analysis, the ontological metaphor of personification, by virtue of the animacy and agentivity features it assigns to pain, gives rise to the understanding of pain by means of a number of interrelated representations and image schematic structure, whereby pain is conceived in socially shared terms. This means that, once perceived as AN ANIMATE AGENT, *ponos* can more easily be represented as being involved in dynamic actions, eventually directed against the patient. Such a construal of the pain experience makes it possible for both the patient and the doctor to establish a channel of communication in order to seek and exchange information about the origin, the properties, and the 'behaviour' of the painful sensation. Hence, it is assumed that, like the objectification metaphor, the ontological metaphor of personification, in addition to being linguistically and conceptually motivated, is also discoursally justified, serving the needs of doctor-patient interaction (see also Lascaratou and Marmaridou, 2005).

8.2.3 The grammaticalisation of *ponos* as subject in transitive structures

The personification of pain as A SELF-WILLED INVASIVE AGENT, AN UNDESIRED, UNINVITED and UNWELCOME VISITOR of the human body ultimately leads to a number of very closely related and interdependent conceptualisations of *ponos*, both reflected in and motivated by its grammaticalisation as the subject of transitive verbs in material processes of 'doing something to someone else'. Not only is *ponos* now grammaticalised as subject, but also its construal is clearly agentive, since it appears in processes of 'doing' where its action is extended to the (sufferer's) self, grammaticalised as direct object. In functional terms, in addition to being the Actor, in these material processes *ponos* is also the Agent, by virtue of its occurrence in effective clauses, i.e. clauses with two participants, where the (sufferer's) self, functioning as Goal, is the other participant.

As the analysis of the data below will show, once established as A SELF-WILLED INTRUSIVE VISITOR of the human body, pain is further understood as AN EXTERNAL INVASIVE ENEMY *setting on* the (sufferer's) self (38)-(40), and as A MALEVOLENT AGGRESSOR, i.e. A RUTHLESS TORTURER acquiring the additional power of *engaging in malevolent, aggressive actions* directed against the (sufferer's) self (41)-(50), hence, as A DYNAMIC AGENTIVE FORCE *holding back* the (sufferer's) self, so as to bring him under its full control and finally *confine* and *imprison* him (51)-(55). (See Peters, 2004: 198–199, for interesting parallels between these Greek metaphors and metaphorical representations of pain in English as evidenced mainly from such adjectival combinations as *pain-afflicted*, *-drawn*, *-shot*, *-stricken*,

-dimmed, *-distorted*, *-worn*, etc. Moreover, for an analysis of Sontag's (1991) account of the understanding of illness – and cancer and AIDS in particular – in terms of invasion by an external to the individual, "an *exogenous* entity to be battled with," see Gwyn, 1999: 205.)

Interestingly, that pain is often metaphorically represented by patients as AN ALIEN INVADER, A DESTROYER threatening to take over and wholly overwhelm the sufferer, is also reported by Aldrich and Eccleston (2000: 1635–1636) in their social constructionist analysis of how sense is made of everyday pain. In one of the most prevalent accounts of this domain of everyday experience, pain is symbolised as "a malign, external and agentic power that is to be feared and avoided at all costs. It threatens identity and can engulf the self, changing it perhaps permanently and for the worse." Remarkably, as will be shown with examples (38)-(40) and even more expressly with (41)-(48), this construal of pain is indeed borne out by the Greek doctor-patient data of this study.

In Lascaratou and Marmaridou (2005), Talmy's force dynamic schema was adopted to interpret those conceptualisations of the painful sensation where *ponos* is grammaticalised as an agentive subject whose action is extended to, or directed at, the (sufferer's) self. It is the presence of these two participants, i.e. *ponos* and the (sufferer's) self, in the same clause and the exploitation of animacy in the ontological metaphor of personification that were assumed to induce such a schematic representation. It was argued that the force dynamic schema, in which two forces – the Agonist and the Antagonist – are represented as interacting, best captures aspects of agentivity and causativity.

Based on our experience of the physical world, and of forces in particular, Talmy's (1988) force dynamic schema applies our naive understanding of the interaction of physical forces to the interaction between two conceptual entities, by conceiving them as force-exerting entities which manifest different, counteracting, force tendencies – namely, toward action or inaction – i.e. as forces bearing different roles as they interact with each other. By mapping the pain experience onto the force image schema, THE (SUFFERER'S) SELF may be construed as the Agonist, i.e. the contestant, confronted with a counteracting force, namely, his PAIN OR THE CAUSE OF HIS PAIN, operating as the Antagonist, i.e. his opponent. As will be shown with new pain metaphors collected in my extensive corpus, this schematic portrayal motivates a number of closely related metaphorical understandings of this domain of human experience.

In the remaining part of this section, I will present an amended version of the initial analysis by systematically associating and contrasting my proposed revised account to Kövecses's (2000) analysis of emotions in general and his related analysis of pain in particular (forth.). To account for emotion metaphors, Kövecses draws on Talmy's (1988) force dynamic schema, i.e. he applies the FORCE schema as the source domain for the extremely general EMOTION IS FORCE 'master metaphor' that he claims to underlie the most well-known metaphors of emotion (e.g. FIRE, OPPONENT, NATURAL FORCE).

To gain a better understanding of how the FORCE schema is applied to emotion metaphors, let us first trace the concept of FORCE as an aspect of the EVENT STRUCTURE metaphor. Thus, within the EVENT STRUCTURE, causes of events are metaphorically seen as forces bringing about changes from one state to another, hence the metaphor CAUSES ARE FORCES. This means that in the EVENT STRUCTURE the causal aspect of events, i.e. causativity, is understood *via* the concept of FORCE. Given that emotions / emotional states are also conceived as having causes, emotions can be metonymically understood in terms of their causes, which gives rise to the metaphor EMOTIONS ARE CAUSES. From these two metaphors the general metaphor EMOTIONS ARE FORCES emerges. Hence, emotions are conceptualised as forces that produce certain (emotional, behavioural, etc.) responses, or effects. Kövecses points out that it is even more natural and obvious for the cause of emotion, i.e. the event or object that gives rise to emotion, to be conceptualised as a cause, and hence as a force, than emotion itself. Yet, it is worth noting here that, as will be discussed more extensively below, the majority of Kövecses's (2000 and forth.) emotion metaphors and a considerable number of his pain metaphors focus on pain / emotion as a force causing external responses rather than on the cause of pain / emotion as a force giving rise to pain / emotion itself.

According to Kövecses (2000: 192), the force schema is systematically mapped onto our conceptualisation of emotion, thus giving rise to our understanding of 'the force of emotion.' He argues (*ibid.*: 61, 85–6, 192) that the source domains of the various specific-level emotion metaphors are all instantiations of the generic concept of force, and therefore, he claims, most of the specific-level metaphors are merely instantiations of a single underlying master metaphor, i.e. the generic-level metaphor EMOTION IS FORCE. In his own words (*ibid.*: 85), "Emotion metaphors are not isolated and unrelated specific-level metaphors, but form a large and intricate system that is organized around the concept of force, as analyzed by Talmy."

For the subsequent discussion of the concept of FORCE in relation to pain, it is crucial to consider the assignment of the force tendencies proposed by Kövecses in his application of the force dynamic schema to the analysis of emotion metaphors (2000: 63), also assumed in his account of the conceptual structure of pain (forth.). Thus, in Kövecses's understanding, the Agonist is typically, though not exclusively, instantiated by the rational self that is or will be emotional, while the Antagonist is instantiated by the cause of emotion / pain or by emotion / pain itself. Moreover, the force tendency toward inaction is assigned to the Agonist (the self), while the force tendency toward action is assigned to the Antagonist (the (cause of) emotion / pain). Hence, the Antagonist exerts force on the Agonist to make it change, i.e.

either to become emotional / to experience pain or to overcome its inaction and produce an external (expressive, physiological, behavioural) action-response, while the Agonist's typical force tendency is to remain unaffected by the Antagonist, i.e. either to remain unemotional / pain-free or to maintain control and refrain from displaying expressive, physiological, or behavioural responses.

At this point it seems useful to compare how the factors in Talmy's force schema are applied in Kövecses's account of emotions and pain and in the present study for the analysis of the Greek pain data, by means of the following table:

Table 1 The force dynamic schema in emotion and pain metaphors

Talmy's force schema	Kövecses's account	Lascaratou's account
Force entities		
Agonist	the rational self	the (sufferer's) self
Antagonist	the (cause of the) emotion / pain	the (cause of the) pain
Intrinsic force tendency		
toward action	Antagonist (emotion)	Antagonist (pain)
toward rest (inaction)	Agonist (self)	Agonist (self)
Resultant of force interaction		
action	self loses control: self is emotional / self responds to emotion	self loses control: self undergoes pain self responds to pain
rest (inaction / stasis)	self maintains control: self remains unemotional self does not respond to emotion	self maintains control: self remains pain-free self does not respond to pain

As it emerges from the Greek doctor-patient data, a different focus is taken by the source domains of the specific-level pain metaphors, as compared to most of Kövecses's (2000 and forth.) emotion and pain metaphors. In particular, it appears that the majority of metaphors employed in the Greek data focus on the cause → force (or cause → emotion / pain) part of the skeletal structure of emotion discussed below, whereas the majority of Kövecses's emotion metaphors and a considerable number of his pain metaphors focus on the force → response (or emotion

/ pain → response) part of the skeletal structure.[10] I will argue that this difference in focus is motivated by the intrinsic character of pain descriptions in doctor-patient interaction which aim basically at highlighting the various forms that the onset of pain takes, as well as the nature, intensity and qualities of the tormenting, confining and immobilising experience, rather than the sufferer's emotional, or other responses. What is more, as I will argue below by proposing an additional assignment of force tendencies (Table 2) to complement the one suggested above (Table 1), there is a salient feature of pain – what I will call a '*meta*-effect' of pain – which differentiates it from most emotions 'proper': while emotions are generally understood as forces internally-motivating external manifestations or action-responses, pain may also appear as an internal force capable of impeding, suppressing or suspending external actions.

To clarify and elaborate these issues, it is necessary to present now the skeletal, yet complete, schema suggested by Kövecses (2000: 85), whereby our basic folk understanding of emotions in terms of forces interacting with each other is captured:

> (1) cause of emotion – force tendency of cause of emotion → (2) self has emotion – force tendency of emotion → (3) self's force tendency ←→ emotion's force tendency → (4) resultant effect

The same folk theory of emotions can be symbolised by means of an even more general schematic representation (Kövecses, *ibid.*: 85; forth.), a simple skeletal scenario which allows the identification of two causal chains, i.e. two complementary parts, more easily:

> cause of emotion → emotion → (controlling emotion) → response

What this skeletal structure essentially captures is that an emotion can be conceived metaphorically both as the effect of a cause, i.e. as a response to a situation, and as the cause of an effect, i.e. of a response:

> cause of emotion → emotion
> (controlling) emotion → response

10. In fact, of the many emotion metaphors that Kövecses (2000) considers, it is basically one which mainly focuses on the cause of emotion, namely the EMOTION IS A PHYSICAL FORCE metaphor and its specific-level metaphors: EMOTION IS A MECHANICAL FORCE, EMOTION IS AN ELECTRIC FORCE, EMOTIONAL EFFECT IS PHYSICAL CONTACT, etc. In his analysis of the conceptual structure of pain (forth.), however, a number of source domains he has proposed as focusing on emotion → response are also suggested as conventional metaphorical source domains focusing on cause of pain → pain, i.e. on the potential causes of pain. More specifically, in addition to PAIN IS A PHYSICAL FORCE, Kövecses (forth.) suggests the metaphors: PAIN IS A CAPTOR / PRISON, PAIN IS A SHARP OBJECT, PAIN IS AN INTRUDER, PAIN IS A TORMENTING ANIMAL, and PAIN IS FIRE / HEAT.

Schematically, these two complementary causal chains show what happens before and after an emotion arises, respectively. While the first part of the scenario represents how the emotion comes about, the second part relates to the ability of emotion to produce effects.

Crucially, for Kövecses, in the causal relationship between emotion and response, the emotion is conceptualised as an action-motivating internal force, and consequently the resulting action-response is understood as the external effect of the internally-motivating emotion force. It appears that it is basically this understanding of emotion force as internally-motivating external actions that underlies the assignment of the tendency toward action to the emotion / pain (Antagonist) in Kövecses's account. Hence, it is natural that metaphors which structure the external behavioural responses / reactions / manifestations of emotions, i.e. those which have to do with the emotion → response causal chain, will be motivated by the assignment of a tendency toward action to the emotion (Antagonist) and of a counteracting tendency toward inaction to the self (Agonist), as suggested by Kövecses.

It seems plausible that in the case of pain the same assignment of force tendencies should be extended to the pain (Antagonist) and the sufferer's self (Agonist), respectively, in relation to the conceptualisation of the external expressive manifestations, physical reactions, and behavioural responses associated with the pain experience. In other words, by virtue of its potential external manifestations, pain may be understood in very similar terms to the ones proposed for the emotions 'proper' with respect to the interaction between the sufferer's self (Agonist) and the pain sensation (Antagonist) in the pain → response causal chain, i.e. the second part of the skeletal structure. Thus, as regards external action-responses, the sufferer's self (Agonist), like the emotional self (Agonist), will attempt to remain inactive and maintain control over its Antagonist, i.e. not engage in action-responses motivated by the force tendency of the pain sensation (Antagonist), such as screaming, crying, whining, weeping, etc. (see section 8.2.4 below).

Moreover, with respect to the onset of pain as captured by the first causal chain (i.e. cause of pain → pain), the analysis of the observed metaphors in the Greek data reveals an understanding of the self (Agonist) and the (cause of) pain (Antagonist) as interacting with the same counteracting force tendencies as in the second causal chain (i.e. pain → response): the (cause of) pain (Antagonist) is the one inclined towards action as its tendency is to produce an unpleasant sensation to the self (Agonist) by counteracting his tendency to remain pain-free.

In our Greek doctor-patient data there is ample empirical evidence that the onset of pain is understood through the conceptualisation of *ponos* as A MALEVOLENT AGGRESSOR SETTING ON THE SELF, expressly represented by (38)-(40). In particular, example (39) portrays both the onset of pain and its exhausting effect, while in (40) the instrument (i.e. a needle) by means of which the self is being acted upon is also profiled:

(38) P: apotoma mja mera *m' epjase enas ponos.*
suddenly one day-ACC I-ACC set-on-PST:3SG a pain-NOM
'Suddenly one day *a pain set on me.*'

(39) P: ama *me pjasi, mu alazi ta fota*!
when I-ACC set-on-PFV:NON-PST:3SG I-GEN change-PRS:3SG the lights-ACC
'When *it sets on me, it wears me out*!'

(40) P: otan *me pjani, veloniazi* ke ponai.
when I-ACC set-on-PRS:3SG pierce (with a needle)-PRS:3SG and hurt-PRS:3SG
'When *it sets on me, it pierces with a needle* and hurts.'

It appears that the Greek data are abundant in what Scarry (1985: 15) calls the "language of agency." The observed metaphorical representation of pain largely conforms to Scarry's claim (*ibid.*: 16) that "the feeling of pain entails the feeling of being acted upon." However, in my corpus this feeling is chiefly expressed in terms of pain itself acting (as a personified entity) on (the sufferer's) self by means of various instruments or weapons, rather than metonymically in terms of specific instruments or weapons pictured as producing pain on their own. Hence, by virtue of its extremely aggressive and frightful actions, pain is further conceptualised as A RUTHLESS TORTURER (see also Lascaratou and Marmaridou, 2005).

Extending the force dynamic schema to this conceptualisation of pain, it is suggested that *ponos* as the Antagonist, i.e. the force counteracting the self-Agonist's tendency to remain pain-free, engages in a variety of aggressive and tormenting activities directed against him, with a view to defeating him and keeping him detained. This is achieved by means of the devastating effect of the various modes of action employed by the *ponos*-Antagonist against the self-Agonist, whereby the variable intensity and qualities of the painful sensation associated with different causes of pain are metonymically understood. Examples (41)-(47) are instantiations of the metaphor PAIN IS A RUTHLESS TORTURER, focusing on various means and forms of torment employed by the TORTURER:

(41) P: *me tarazi* olo, olo, apo ton pono *me tinazi* olo eδo, *varai* etsi me kati *bixtes*...
I-ACC agitate-PRS:3SG all all by the pain-ACC I-ACC shake-PRS:3SG all here strike-PRS:3SG like-this with some thrusts-ACC
'*It agitates me*, all over, *I am shaken*, all over here by pain, *it strikes* (*me*) as if *it were thrusting* (*me*)...'

(42) P: ...endonos ponos ke *me xtipuse* os to γonato kato.
intense pain-NOM and I-ACC beat-IPFV:3SG as-far-as the knee-ACC below
'...an intense pain and *it beat me* further down as far as my knee.'

(43) P: tora, as pume, *me kei me kei.*
now let's say-PFV:NON-PST:1PL I-ACC burn-PRS:3SG I-ACC burn-PRS:3SG
'Now, for instance, *it's burning me, it's burning me.*'

(44) P: *mja floya m'angiloni… me tsimbai, me troi.*
a flame-NOM I-ACC sting-PRS:3SG I-ACC prick-PRS:3SG I-ACC consume-PRS:3SG
'*A flame is stinging me… it is pricking me, it is consuming me.*'

(45) D: *sas tsimbai* to vraδi *o ponos*?
you-ACC prick-PRS:3SG the night-ACC the pain-NOM
'*Does the pain prick you* at night?'

P: uu, afu xθes to vraδi δen borusa na kimiθo.
ooh since yesterday the night-ACC not can-IPFV:1SG to-PARTCL sleep-PFV:NON-PST:1SG
'Oh yeah, imagine last night I couldn't sleep.'

(46) D: ke ponate?
and hurt-PRS:2PL
'And do you suffer pain?'

P: e afu *me… pniji.*
eh since I-ACC strangle-PRS:3SG
'Eh, since *it… strangles me.*'

D: *sas sfingi* δilaδi.
you-ACC:PL squeeze-PRS:3SG that-is
'*It squeezes you*, that is.'

P: *me sfingi.*
I-ACC squeeze-PRS:3SG
'*It squeezes me.*'

(47) P: …arxizi ke *me travai…* apo δo ke pera.
start-PRS:3SG and I-ACC pull-PRS:3SG from here and away
'…indeed it starts *pulling me…* from this point.'

D: *traviyma* njoθete eδo.
pull-ACC feel-PRS:2PL here
'*It's a sensation of pulling* that you have here.'

P: ne. alote *afto*, kserete, *travai…* ke *xtipai* ke eδo, eno alote *travai* mono eδo ke *δe xtipai* ke kato.
yes sometimes this know-PRS:2PL pull-PRS:3SG and beat-PRS:3SG and here while sometimes pull-PRS:3SG only here and not beat-PRS:3SG and below
'Yes. Sometimes *this*, you know, *pulls…* and *beats* here too, while sometimes *it* only *pulls* here and *it doesn't beat* below.'

(48) P: perna *enas ponos*… ke *me sfazi*.
pass-PRS:3SG a pain-NOM and I-ACC slaughter-PRS:3SG
'*A pain* passes… and *slaughters me*.'

If we look at these extracts more thoroughly, we observe that the potential or actual tissue damage experienced by the self is represented as being caused by A VICIOUS TORTURER exerting force which is felt as *piercing* (40), *agitating* (41), *shaking* (41), *striking* (41), *thrusting* (41), *beating* (42) and (47), *burning* (43) and (44), *stinging* (44), *pricking* (44) and (45), *consuming* (44), *strangling* (46), *squeezing* (46), and *pulling* (47). Finally, if the tissue damage is sensed as being *slaughtering*, i.e. as if produced with the use of a penetrating sharp-bladed, cutting knife, like those employed for slaughtering animals or human beings, an understanding of pain as A SLAUGHTERER using such a knife may arise, as shown in (34), repeated here under (48). It is worth noting at this point that the focusing of this metaphor on the first causal chain (i.e. cause of pain → pain) of the scenario, is motivated by the semantic structure of the particular verb *sfazo* 'to slaughter', by virtue of the use of a sharp-bladed, cutting instrument that it entails,[11] while, as we shall see below, the verb *skotono* 'to kill', which simply means 'to put to death' without entailing the use of any specific instrument, is used in metaphors focusing on the second causal chain (i.e. pain → response / effect).

Thus, the causes of pain – the actual or potential tissue damage – are metonymically conceptualised as the instruments of torment or forces employed by the PAIN AS A RUTHLESS TORTURER OF SLAUGHTERER (Antagonist) and they include PHYSICAL AGITATION, PHYSICAL FORCE, MECHANICAL FORCE, SWORD / DAGGER / SHARP OBJECT, STING, SHARP POINT(S), NEEDLE, and SLAUGHTERER'S KNIFE, giving rise to the metaphors:

PAIN IS PHYSICAL AGITATION

(41) *me tarazi* olo, olo, apo ton pono *me tinazi* olo eδo
'*it agitates me*, all over, *I am shaken*, all over here by pain'

PAIN IS A PHYSICAL FORCE / A MECHANICAL FORCE

(41) *varai*
'*it strikes (me)*'

(42) *endonos ponos* ke *me xtipuse* os to γonato kato
'*an intense pain* and *it beat me* further down as far as my knee'

11. The suggested interpretation is further supported by the non-technical pain descriptor *sfaχtis*, literally 'slaughterer', a term commonly used to describe penetrating and intense pain, chiefly back pain, low back pain, or pain in the ribs.

(46) e afu *me... pniji*
'eh, since *it... strangles me*'
me sfingi
'*it squeezes me*'

(47) arxizi ke *me travai*... apo δo ke pera
'indeed *it* starts *pulling me*... from this point'
traviyma njoθete eδo
'*it's a sensation of pulling* that you have here'
alote *afto*, kserete, *travai*... ke *xtipai* ke eδo, eno alote *travai* mono eδo ke *δe xtipai* ke kato
'sometimes *this*, you know, *pulls*... and *beats* here too, while sometimes *it* only *pulls* here and *it* doesn't *beat* below'

PAIN IS A NEEDLE

(40) *veloniazi* ke ponai
'*it pierces with a needle* and hurts'

PAIN IS A SWORD / DAGGER / SHARP OBJECT

(41) *varai* etsi me kati *bixtes*
'*it strikes* (*me*) as if it *were thrusting* (*me*)'

PAIN IS A STING

(44) mja floγa *m'angiloni*
'a flame is *stinging me*'

PAIN IS (A) SHARP POINT(S)

(44) *me tsimbai*
'*it is pricking me*'

(45) sas *tsimbai* to vraδi *o ponos*?
'does *the pain prick you* at night?'

PAIN IS FIRE / HEAT

(43) *me kei, me kei*
'*it's burning me, it's burning me*'

(44) *mja floγa* m'angiloni
'*a flame* is stinging me'

PAIN IS A SLAUGHTERER'S KNIFE

(48) perna *enas ponos*... ke *me sfazi*
'*a pain* passes... and *slaughters me*'

To gain a better understanding of the conceptual mechanisms involved here, it is important to realise that the source domains of the specific-level metaphors presented above, i.e. the various types of (actual or potential) tissue damage causing various types of painful sensation, are derived through a metonymic process. From the analysis of the Greek data, it appears that the general metonymic relationship INSTRUMENT / MEANS FOR ACTION / EVENT forms the metonymic basis of the causes of pain: a variety of instruments or forces (e.g. SWORD / DAGGER / SHARP OBJECT, STING, SHARP POINT(S), NEEDLE, SLAUGHTERER'S KNIFE, FIRE / HEAT, PHYSICAL AGITATION, PHYSICAL FORCE, and MECHANICAL FORCE) stand for different types of pain-inducing tissue damage that they may produce. Hence, the metonymic vehicle (the instrument / means / force whereby mental access to the tissue damage is provided) subsequently becomes the source domain for the metaphorical conceptualisation of the painful experience (see also Kövecses, forth.), e.g. the understanding of the experience of pain as one with (i.e. *caused by*) a sharp object. Thus, the force of pain with its variable intensity and qualities is metaphorically conceptualised in terms of a range of metonymically derived (physical) causes, giving rise to the metaphors above. I will argue that this metonymic basis of the metaphorical conceptualisation of the causes of pain is very crucial.

In the light of Kövecses's (2000: 164–5, 185, 190–1 and forth.) sense of 'embodiment' proposed for emotions (already discussed above in section 8.2.2), I suggest that the collected Greek pain metaphors focusing on the causes of pain are constrained by, i.e. they cannot contradict, the universal aspects of the body's physiological functioning in the experience of pain. To put this in simple words, assuming that the human body has a universal physiology, it is reasonable to further presume that the physical aspect of pain, namely, the particular types of tissue damage with their accompanying sensory effects, are also universal. This assumed universality of human physiology in pain is hypothesised to motivate, i.e. impose constraints on, the way human beings view their bodies and their physiological functioning in pain. Hence, it seems sensible to suggest that the cognitive mechanisms (conceptual metonymies and metaphors) involved in understanding this domain of human experience are also constrained by universal aspects of human physiology, potentially giving rise to similar linguistic realisations across languages. In particular, metonymy being a widely used cognitive process whereby mental access to a conceptual entity is provided *via* another conceptual entity within the same domain, it is assumed that comparable metonymically derived metaphorical (conceptual and linguistic) representations of the sensory aspect of the pain experience in terms of its causes (the actual or potential tissue damage) will be observed cross-linguistically or even near-universally.[12]

Evidence that these assumptions are largely justifiable does not come only from the analysis of pain metaphors in other languages, such as Kövecses (forth.)

12. One could perhaps venture to suggest that these expressions are so much constrained by universal physiology that they are very close to depicting how the various forms of tissue damage are literally experienced by the sufferer.

where a number of metonymically derived metaphors are proposed for English, some of which are related to the ones observed in the Greek data, e.g. PAIN IS A SHARP OBJECT, PAIN IS FIRE / HEAT, PAIN IS A TORMENTING ANIMAL, etc. Most importantly, the majority of extensively used conventionalised pain descriptors, included in such widely applied assessment tools as the McGill Pain Questionnaire and its translations in many languages, are metaphorical in nature, their emergence involving the metonymic process discussed above. To mention but a few of the 78 terms employed in the MPQ, pain is described as *beating*, *shooting*, *stabbing*, *flashing*, *burning*, *scalding*, *stinging*, *gnawing*, and *splitting*.

It is precisely by virtue of the constraints imposed by universal physiology on the metaphorical conceptualisation of pain that metaphorically structured pain descriptors and terms acquire their diagnostic value. In other words, if the (near-) universal physical aspects of pain, i.e. sensory effects metonymically conceptualised in terms of particular types of tissue damage, motivate and constrain the metaphorical representation of pain, it is hypothesised that the identification of the type of tissue damage should be facilitated by the use of constrained conceptual and linguistic metaphors. For example, if the tissue damage produces a sensation of pricking, the concept SHARP OBJECT may be applied metonymically and give rise to the metaphor PAIN IS A SHARP OBJECT. If, as assumed, the structuring of pain provided by this metaphor does not contradict the aspects of physiology associated with the particular quality of pain, then in turn the metaphor should potentially make it easier to identify the type of damage causing that pain.

Let us now move on to the second causal chain (i.e. pain → response) of the scenario, i.e. what happens after pain is produced, in relation to its ability to make the sufferer's self react.

With respect to external physiological, behavioural and expressive pain responses, e.g. throbbing, groaning, crying, screaming, whining, weeping, etc., as was pointed out above, we observe that such reactions are not highlighted in the effective material processes where *ponos* is an Actor / Agent participant that were collected in the Greek doctor-patient data of the present study. (See, however 8.2.4 for a discussion of the construal of *ponos* as a circumstance of cause bringing about such external responses.) It is mainly some of the psychological effects of pain that are metaphorically structured in such two-participant clauses. Thus, for example, the concept of MADNESS / INSANITY – regularly applied to represent severe pain intensity (see (23) and (24) above) – is also applied with respect to the distressing psychological effects of intense pain, giving rise to the metaphor BEING IN PAIN IS BEING INSANE, as shown in (49):

(49) R: *i poni tis mesis ton exun trelani.*
the pains-NOM the low-back-GEN he-ACC have-PRS:3PL madden-PFV
'*His low back pains have driven him crazy.*'

What is more, if the sufferer's self-Agonist is completely overcome by the devastating force of the pain-Antagonist to the point that he feels as if he has ceased to live, an understanding of pain as A KILLER may arise (50):

(50) P: ax, me ponai, *me skotoni.*
ouch I-ACC hurt-PRS:3SG I-ACC kill-PRS:3SG
'Ouch, it's hurting me, *it's killing me.*'

What seems to me to clearly emerge from the exploration of the doctor-patient dialogues is what, in my understanding, appears to be one of the most salient features of the pain experience taken as a whole and in particular of chronic pain, namely, the paralysing and confining effect that it may have on the (sufferer's) self. On the basis of the data analysis and my intuitions deriving from my personal experience, I will venture to suggest that the paralysing and confining feelings often experienced by the (sufferer's) self at the various stages of the painful condition can be conceived as a *meta*-effect of pain. What I am trying to suggest by using this characterisation is that this type of inner reaction (often, but not necessarily, arising from the sufferer's literal, i.e. physical, immobilisation / confinement) should be identified with the *existence* of pain overall, as an *accompanying feature* rather than strictly speaking as *an effect* of the painful experience. Hence, I do not see it as being exclusively related with any of the two major causal chains (i.e. cause → pain or pain → response). Moreover, I assume that this sense of immobilisation or imprisonment may be experienced by the self independently of whether the self does or does not display external responses.

This sense of IMPRISONMENT or CONFINING EXPERIENCE emerging from the Greek data, whereby the person in pain feels trapped with a private reality, essentially coincides with Kugelmann's (1999: 1671) view that pain is "the perimeter of existential place," which suggests that pain itself is "a boundary, a limitation."[13] Seen from that angle, the metaphorical understanding of *ponos* as IMPRISONMENT or CONFINEMENT could be associated with the very general metaphor EXISTENCE OF EMOTION IS BEING IN A BOUNDED SPACE, applying to all emotion concepts (e.g. *she is in love*, *ime se foveri ayonia* 'I am in terrible suspense', *imaste se paniko* 'we are in panic', *ime se meyali apelpisia*, 'I am in great despair').[14]

Let us observe this understanding of *ponos* in the following examples:

(51) P: *δe m'afini* (o ponos) na sikoθo.
not I-ACC let-PRS:3SG (the pain-NOM) to-PARTCL get-up-PFV:NON-PST:1SG
'*It* (the pain) *does not let me* stand up.'

(52) P: *aftos o iδjos ponos* meγaloni ke *δe m'afini.*
this the same pain-NOM grow-PRS:3SG and not I-ACC let-PRS:3SG
'*This very same pain* grows and *doesn't let go of me.*'

(53) D: δen exete tin psixolojiki δjaθesi na kanete praγmata ke nomizete oti *o ponos sas emboδizi.*
not have-PRS:2PL the psychological mood-ACC to-PARTCL do-PRS:2PL things-ACC and think-PRS:2PL that the pain-NOM you-ACC prevent-PRS:3SG
'You are not in the mood to do things and you think that it is *the pain* that *prevents you.*'

(54) D: to vraδi *δe s'afini* na kimiθis?
the night-ACC not you-ACC let-PRS:3SG to-PARTCL sleep-PFV:NON-PST:2SG
'*Doesn't it let you* sleep at night?'

---

13. Kugelmann observes that, in addition to being described as A CONFINEMENT, symbolically as A PRISON, pain is also depicted as a kind of HOMELESSNESS. He points out that both are related by a common element, namely, that in both instances, "the person is cut off from the possibility of dwelling, of being at home." He suggests that PRISON and HOMELESSNESS are "two contemporary versions of the poorhouse of earlier times", both representing INDIGENCE. In the light of this view, the following extract from our data, uttered by an elderly patient while she was experiencing excruciating pain following orthopaedic surgery, could be interpreted as an instance of such a feeling of INDIGENCE:

P: a, re *kurelu*! *kurelu*! imun perifani s' aftin tin ilikia… ke *ejina kurelu*…
oh you ragged-woman-VOC ragged-woman-VOC be-PST:1SG at this the age-ACC and become-PST:1SG ragged-woman-NOM
'Oh, my! Look at me! *A ragged woman*! *A ragged woman*! I used to be proud at that age… and *I've become a ragged woman*…'

14. Peters (2004: 199) interprets the English pattern *to be in pain* as an instantiation of the metaphor PAIN IS A CONTAINER.

(55) D: exete kapja δrastiriotita… i *o ponos sas exi periorisi sto spiti…?*
have-PRS:2PL some activity-ACC or the pain-NOM you-ACC have-PRS:3SG confine-PFV in-the house-ACC
'Do you have any activity… or has the pain *confined you at home…?*'

In (51) *ponos* is construed as obstructing the sufferer's motion, in (52) as holding him back, in (53) as impeding his everyday activity and punishing him by depriving him of the ability and right to sleep (54), and in (55) as confining him at home.

It is, therefore, the resultant effect of the pain-Antagonist's counter-acting force which motivates the rendering of *ponos* as A DYNAMIC AGENTIVE FORCE *holding back* the self (51)-(55) so as to bring him under its full control and finally immobilise, confine and detain him, as AN IMPRISONING ENEMY (55). It follows, therefore, that the interpretation of such pain metaphors observed in the Greek data calls for a different assignment of force tendencies in terms of Talmy's force dynamic image schema.

Hence, along the lines of Lascaratou and Marmaridou (2005), the entity that is inclined towards action is taken to be THE (SUFFERER'S) SELF construed as the Agonist, while the force tendency toward inaction (stasis) is assigned to *ponos*, i.e. the PAIN construed as the Antagonist. Therefore, the Agonist's force tendency is to counteract the Antagonist's immobilising and confining tendency and maintain his ability to act and move, while the Antagonist's characteristic force tendency is to hold back the Agonist, by obstructing his activity and motion. If the pain-Antagonist's immobilising force counteracts the self-Agonist's inclination towards action, then the latter will typically become inactive. Thus, by virtue of the causative implications involved in this schematic structure, PAIN appears as a prototypical Agent exerting power over THE (SUFFERER'S) SELF with a view to neutralising him.

Let us illustrate schematically the proposed different assignment of force tendencies and contrast it to our initial application of Talmy's force schema figuring in Table 1:

I suggest that this different assignment of force tendencies, in relation to what I intuitively consider to be a salient feature of pain, captures an essential difference between pain and the majority of emotions 'proper'. It appears that, by virtue of its emotional aspect and with respect to the conceptualisation of its outward manifestations, pain is comparable to most emotions, which are generally viewed as forces internally-motivating external actions. On the other hand, pain is understood as an internal, potentially paralysing force, i.e. one that may impede, suppress or suspend external actions. However, in relation to the paralysing effect of pain, I would presume that some of the negatively evaluated emotions, such as fear, sadness, depression, etc. could also be analysed along these lines.

Table 2 The force dynamic schema in metaphors of the '*meta*-effect' of pain

Talmy's force schema	**Lascaratou's account**	
	Cause → Pain → **Pain → External Response**	**Pain = Imprisonment / Immobilisation**
Force entities		
Agonist	the (sufferer's) self	the (sufferer's) self
Antagonist	the (cause of the) pain	the (cause of the) pain
Intrinsic force tendency		
toward action	Antagonist (pain)	Agonist (self)
toward rest (inaction)	Agonist (self)	Antagonist (pain)
Resultant of force interaction		
action	self loses control: self undergoes pain self responds to pain	self maintains control: self remains active
rest (inaction / stasis)	self maintains control: self remains pain-free self does not respond to pain	self loses control: self becomes inactive

8.2.4 The construal of *ponos* as circumstance of cause

Parallel to the conceptualisation of *ponos* as AN ANIMATE AGENTIVE TORTURER, there appears its metaphorical construal as a torture-like experience. Consider the following, where the painful sensation is likened to AN AGONISING TRAGEDY, A TORTURE or TORMENT:

(56) P: to vraδi ine to *δrama*, to vraδi ine to *δrama*.
the night-ACC be-PRS:3SG the tragedy-NOM the night-ACC be-PRS:3SG the tragedy-NOM
'At night it is *a tragedy*, at night it is *a tragedy*.'

(57) P: *ine vasanistirio* to prama.
be-PRS:3SG torture the thing-NOM
'The whole thing is *a torture*.'

Departing from material effective processes where *ponos* is the Actor / Agent, we move on to clauses profiling *ponos* mainly as a circumstance of cause rather than as a participant. This circumstantial construal of *ponos* is primarily marked by its co-occurrence with the preposition *apo* 'from', clearly denoting cause, and secondarily with the preposition *se* 'in', also used to denote cause. Hence, the understanding of *ponos* as a condition under which the sufferer is tormented and forced to lose control by displaying various external responses, is reflected in and motivated by its grammatical construal as a circumstance of cause. Therefore, the representation of pain as a forceful cause deriving from the very general metaphor CAUSES ARE FORCES discussed above (section 8.2.3), underlies the conceptualisation of pain as a TORMENTOR / TORTURER instantiated in the following examples:

(58) P: *ksipnao apo tus ponus.*
wake-up-PRS:1SG from-the pains-ACC
'*I wake up from the pains.*'

(59) D: θes na... *oriese ston pono?*
want-PRS:2SG to-PARTCL scream-PRS:2SG in-the pain-ACC
'*Do you want to... scream from (the) pain?*'

(60) P: *δangono ta siδera apo tus ponus.*
bite-PRS:1SG the irons-ACC from-the pains-ACC
'*My pains make me feel like biting on iron.*'

(61) P: *lipoθimisa apo ton pono.*
faint-PST:1SG from-the pain-ACC
'*I fainted from (the) pain.*'

(62) P: *peθeno stus ponus.*
die-PRS:1SG in-the pains-ACC
'*I die from the pains.*'

(63) P: po po! katse. *peθana!*
tut tut sit-IMP:2SG die-PST:1SG
'My goodness! Just wait. *I'm dead!*'

It is worth noting that the metaphors observed in the data above focus on the force → response (pain → response) part of the skeletal structure of pain, unlike the ones we have examined so far, which have to do with the cause → force (or cause → pain) part of the structure. As argued earlier (section 8.2.3), the metaphorical representations of pain which focus on the causal relationship between pain and its potential external expressive, physical, and behavioural responses may be paralleled to the metaphors which structure the emotion → response causal chain. In other words, like emotion in general, pain here is understood as a force, a forceful cause, internally-motivating external actions on the part of the sufferer. It seems, therefore, reasonable to suggest that, in such metaphorical representations of external pain reactions, the interaction between the sufferer's self (Agonist) and the pain sensation (Antagonist) may be understood in very similar terms to the ones proposed for the emotions 'proper', with respect to their force tendencies: a tendency toward action will be assigned to pain (Antagonist) and a counteracting tendency toward inaction to the self (Agonist). This means that, like the emotional self (Agonist), the sufferer's self (Agonist), will attempt to remain inactive, i.e. counteract his pain-Antagonist's force tendency toward action and maintain control over it. Loss of control on the part of the sufferer's self will lead to external action-responses, such as the ones illustrated in the data, e.g. *waking up in one's sleep* (58), *screaming* (59), '*biting on iron*' (60), *fainting* (61) or (*feeling like*) *dying* (62) and (63).

Thus, our material confirms the observation put forward by Söderberg and Norberg (1995: 58) that dramatic and very negative metaphorical expressions used by patients indicate that they see themselves as victims of the pain experience. This feeling of victimisation experienced by the patient may evoke in him the sentiment that his pain is a condition, a circumstance from which he cannot escape and which, therefore, he must learn to live with:

(64) D: emaθes *na zis me ton pono su.*
learn-PST:2SG to-PARTCL live-PRS:2SG with the pain-ACC your
'You have learnt *to live with your pain*.'

Alternatively, the self-Agonist may refuse to accept his pain-Antagonist and develop resistance against his condition:

(65) P: *ime skliri ston pono.*
be-PRS:1SG tough in-the pain-ACC
'*I'm tough with pain*.'

8.2.5 The grammaticalisation of *ponos* as object in transitive structures

The resistance developed by the sufferer's self, which may take on various forms, is reflected in and motivated by the grammaticalisation of *ponos* as object of transitive verbs denoting attempt at active control or passive opposition on the part of the sufferer's self grammaticalised as subject. In functional terms, this means that the roles of the sufferer's self and his pain are now reversed: it is the sufferer's self which is profiled as the Actor / Agent, i.e. 'the doer of the deed', in material effective processes where *ponos* is 'demoted' to Goal, i.e. the entity to which the sufferer's action is extended. Despite this reversal of grammatical functions and participant roles, the painful experience can still be mapped onto the force dynamic schema, the sufferer's self and *ponos* retaining their roles of Agonist inclined toward motion and Antagonist having a counteracting force tendency, respectively.

The following examples illustrate the understanding of the sufferer's self and his pain as opponents in a struggle, hence giving rise to the metaphor PAIN IS AN OPPONENT that must be *set under control* or be *endured* at all costs. The sufferer's self (Agonist) is engaged in an attempt to defeat his pain-Antagonist by maintaining control over its force which counteracts his own activity. Thus, the suffering Agonist's efforts materialise either as ACTIVE CONTROL exerted over the painful sensation (67), or as mere PASSIVE OPPOSITION (68) in the case that he fails to maintain active control over pain without, however, entirely giving in to his opponent either.

(66) P: epitelus, δose mu kati, *δen andexo tus ponus.*
at-last give-IMP:2SG I-GEN something not stand-PRS:1SG the pains-ACC
'For goodness sake, give me something, *I can't stand the pains.*'

(67) P: *exo θesi ipo elenxo… tus ponus*, iparxi ke kapja veltiosi me to voltaren.
have-PRS:1SG get-PFV under control-ACC the pains-ACC exist-PRS:3SG and some improvement-NOM with the voltaren
'*I have got the pains under control*, there is even some improvement with Voltaren.'

(68) D: *tin karδia petra* ke θa *ipomenume ton pono.*
the heart-ACC stone-ACC and will endure-PRS:1PL the pain-ACC
'We shall turn *our hearts into stones* so as *to endure the pain.*'

Control being one of the very general dimensions of experience, along with existence, intensity, passivity, difficulty, harm, etc. (see section 8.2.2 above), various metaphors within the EVENT STRUCTURE metaphor, and the FORCE metaphor, in particular, are used to highlight it, e.g. the general metaphor ATTEMPT AT CONTROL IS STRUGGLE WITH FORCE. In the domain of emotions the specific-level metaphor takes the form ATTEMPT AT EMOTIONAL CONTROL IS TRYING TO OVERCOME AN OPPONENT, which underlies the conceptualisation of the rational self and emotions as opponents in a struggle whereby the self tries to maintain emotional control, instantiated in the metaphor EMOTION IS AN OPPONENT (see Kövecses, 2000: 42–4, 68–69, 193). The concept of emotional control is essentially present in all emotion metaphors, e.g. EMOTION IS A WILD ANIMAL / A PHYSICAL FORCE / A MENTAL FORCE / A SOCIAL SUPERIOR, etc. The fact that control as a central issue in the conceptualisation of emotions is reflected in many emotion metaphors is also suggested by Kidron and Kuzar (2002: 130).

Ultimately, the ontological metaphor of personification motivates the representation of *ponos* as AN ANGRY DEITY whose favour the patient struggles to win. This is very vividly conveyed in the following humorous dialogue where the sufferer wonders how he may *propitiate* his pain and his interlocutor responds playfully by proposing to bless the suffering leg!

(69) P: ...pos na *ton eksileoso*?
how to-PARTCL it-ACC propitiate-PFV:NON-PST:1SG
'...how *could I propitiate it*?'
D: *ton pono θa ton eksileosis*? tora. *θa* to... *θa* to *evlojiso* eγo to poδi ke θa *to eksileosume.*
the pain-ACC will it-ACC propitiate-PFV:NON-PST:2SG now will it-ACC will it-ACC bless-PFV:NON-PST:1SG I-NOM the leg-ACC and will it-ACC propitiate-PFV:NON-PST:1PL
'Do you wish *to propitiate the pain*? Now. *I will... I will bless* the leg and *we will propitiate it*.'

By controlling, enduring and propitiating pain, the patient-Agonist aims at safeguarding his body against his Antagonist's attack or invasion. The body, remaining "a dominant metaphor and model for self" (Aldrich and Eccleston, 2000: 1632), provides defensible boundaries that must be protected, against pain's intrinsic ability to change and disassemble self (*ibid.*: 1640).

Finally, if the suffering Agonist achieves his ultimate goal, which is to get rid of his painful condition, the *ponos*-Antagonist will eventually RETREAT (70) and (71) or, taking the most hopeful view, will be entirely DEFEATED. Example (72) is an instance of the sufferer's triumphant reaction following his victory over the enemy.

(70) P: *ipoxorise* kapos, *ipoxorise.*
subside-PST:3SG somewhat subside-PST:3SG
'*It has subsided* to some extent, *it has subsided*.'

(71) D: sas exi *ipoxorisi* me to aftokolito?
you-GEN:PL have-PRS:3SG subside-PFV with the self-adhesive-ACC
'*Has it subsided* with the adhesive patch?'

(72) D: bravo su, afto itan!
well-done you-GEN this-NOM be-PST:3SG
'Congratulations to you, that was it!'
P: *nikisa*!
win-PST:1SG
'*I've won!*'

8.3 Lost for words

As was already discussed in the introductory section on metaphor and pain, the use of metaphorical pain language by patients is an indication that they have trouble in describing their pain experience explicitly, due to its subjective character and complexity. This difficulty sometimes becomes insurmountable and results in actual loss of words. In particular, this is most commonly observed among chronic pain patients, who may be unable to provide explicit descriptions of pain, despite their constant, yet often vaguely phrased complaints (Borsook, LeBel and McPeek, 1998: 452). This observation is also attested in DeSouza and Frank's (2000: 212) study on the subjectivity of the painful sensation experienced by people suffering from chronic back pain, where it is equally interpreted as reflecting their inability "to put words to their pain experience." Patients' difficulty in verbalising their sensory experiences as witnessed in Söderberg and Norberg (1995: 57–58) is further supported by Hallberg and Carlsson (2000: 32), who point out that "difficulty in finding words to express feelings (alexithymia)[15] has been reported as a characteristic in psychosomatic patients."[16]

Loss of words on the part of chronic pain patients is confirmed in our doctor-patient dialogues, where some very interesting instances are observed. Thus, patients sometimes simply declare their inability to verbalise, describe or define their painful condition, e.g. (73) and (74), without actually being in a position to provide a particular reason. Their desperate efforts to articulate their inner suffering are more dramatically revealed in those recurring cases, such as (75) and (77), where the patients, when asked to describe their pain, respond by reversing the question to their interlocutor, as if he were more capable of providing a pain description on their behalf. Even though this is not always explicitly stated like in dialogues (76) and (77), it seems that in chronic pain patients loss of words primarily derives from

15. Though the term 'alexithymia' is very attractive and I initially intended to adopt it in this discussion, I finally decided not to do so because of the ambiguity deriving from its two potential interpretations. As Tzavaras (1999: 243) explains in a footnote, this term was introduced by the Greek-American psychiatrist-psychoanalyst Peter Sifneos, whose explicit intention was to create a neologism so as to refer to the dys-connectionist concept 'depriving words from the possibility of denoting one's feelings.' To that end, he made up a morphologically complex word form to signify 'expressing one's feelings verbally', by putting together *lexi / leksi* 'word' and *thymia* 'feelings', and then he attached the negative Greek prefix *a-* before it to produce the intended negative meaning. However, the sequence *alexi / aleksi-* is also a prefix by itself, meaning 'protect' or 'repel', which is quite productive and occurs in the name *aleksanδros* 'Alexander' and in such words as *aleksi-piros* 'fireproof' *aleksi-keravno* 'lightning-conductor'. Hence, if 'alexithymia' is analysed as *alexi-thymia* rather than the originally intended *a-lexi-thymia*, it comes to mean 'repelling or protecting one's feelings', which is, of course quite different. Apparently, Hallberg and Carlsson (2000), use the term with Sifneos's original semantic content. To be honest, it seems to me that it is precisely the ambiguity involved in the term that makes it so appealing.

16. Though, loss of words may be observed in relation to more or less all emotional experiences, what makes it worth noting with respect to pain is the fact that pain has so many properties in terms of which it may be identified, e.g. temporal location and extent, variable location within the body, intensity and diverse qualities.

their intense involvement in the pain experience resulting from their long-lasting familiarisation with it. Hence, pain becomes so much part of themselves that they cannot gain the necessary distance that would enable them to describe it.

(73) P: *δen boro na ton periγrapso* ti ponos, *δen boro na ton periγrapso.*
not can-PRS:1SG to-PARTCL it-ACC describe-PFV:NON-PST:1SG what pain-ACC not can-PRS:1SG to-PARTCL it-ACC describe-PFV:NON-PST:1SG
'*I can't describe it*, what kind of pain it is, *I can't describe it.*'

(74) P: *δen boro na oriso* ton pono, na san zoon kano. na, *na ekfrasto* ti njoθo.
not can-PRS:1SG to-PARTCL define-PFV:NON-PST:1SG the pain-ACC here like animal-ACC do-PRS:1SG to to-PARTCL express-PFV:NON-PST:1SG what feel-PRS:1SG
'*I can't define* the pain, look, I behave like an animal. I can't express what I feel.'

(75) D: ke pos in' aftos o ponos?
and how be-PRS:3SG this the pain-NOM
'And what is this pain like?'

P: tora, *kseris esi pos ine o ponos. pos ine o ponos kseris esi.*
now know-PRS:2SG you-NOM how be-PRS:3SG the pain-NOM how be-PRS:3SG the pain-NOM know-PRS:2SG you-NOM
'Now, *you know what the pain is like. What the pain is like, you are the one to know.*'

D: e?
what
'What?'

P: *pos ine o ponos kseris esi. pos ine o ponos kseris esi.*
how be-PRS:3SG the pain-NOM know-PRS:2SG you-NOM how be-PRS:3SG the pain-NOM know-PRS:2SG you-NOM
'*What the pain is like, you are the one to know. What the pain is like, you are the one to know.*'

D: oxi, δen ksero eγo. esi kseris, esi. pos ine o ponos, δilaδi? pos ton njoθis afton ton pono? ti?
no not know-PRS:1SG I-NOM you-NOM know-PRS:2SG you-NOM how be-PRS:3SG the pain-NOM that-is how it-ACC feel-PRS:2SG this the pain-ACC what
'No, I am not the one to know. You are the one to know. You. That is, what is the pain like? How do you feel this pain?'

P: δen ipoferete.
not tolerate-PASS:PRS:3SG
'It's intolerable.'

(76) P: *exo* kata kapjo tropo *mja eksikiosi* afti ti stiɣmi ke… *δen ime se θesi na sas periɣrapso* me poli safinia *jati ine mja katastasi makroxronia.*
have-PRS:1SG in some way a familiarisation-ACC this the moment-ACC and not be-PRS:1SG in position-ACC to-PARTCL you-GEN:PL describe-PFV:NON-PST:1SG with much explicitness-ACC because be-PRS:3SG a situation long-lasting-NOM
'*I have*, in a sense, *some familiarisation* at present and… *I'm not in a position to describe* (it) *to you* very explicitly *because it's been a long-lasting situation*.'

(77) D: orea, pos ton periɣrafis afto ton pono?
right-ADV how it-ACC describe-PRS:2SG this the pain-ACC
'Right, how do you describe this pain?'

P: *periɣrapse ton esi.*
describe-IMP:2SG it-ACC you-NOM
'*You describe it*.'

D: eɣo? eɣo δen ponao oxtomisi mines.
I-NOM I-NOM not hurt-PRS:1SG eight-and-a-half months-ACC
'Me? It's not me who's been in pain for eight and a half months.'

P: oxtomisi mines eɣo ponao.
eight-and-a-half months-ACC I-NOM hurt-PRS:1SG
'It's me who's been in pain for eight and a half months.'

D: pos ton esθanese re peδi mu, san ti, ti? δos' tu ena epiθeto.
how it-ACC feel-PRS:2SG man my like what what give-IMP:2SG it-GEN an adjective-ACC
'How does it feel, man, like what, what? Give it a name.'

P: *ton siniθisa.*
it-ACC got-used-to-PST:1SG
'*I've got used to it*.'

D: ena prozδiorizmo δos' tu.
an attribute-ACC give-IMP:2SG it-GEN
'Characterise it.'

P: *ton siniθisa*, su leo.
it-ACC got-used-to-PST:1SG you-GEN tell-PRS:1SG
'I'm telling you, *I've got used to it*.'

8.4 Concluding remarks

The analysis of *ponos* nominal constructions from a cognitive semantics perspective with data drawn from the extensive material of this study has once more brought out the close relation between cognition and linguistic structure. Hence, the pain-related data constitute empirical evidence in support of the assumption that linguistic choices (e.g. the selection of particular lexical frames and the linguistic realisation of metaphors) are motivated by image schematic conceptual structure, and, at the same time, everyday experience is construed in terms of conceptualisations, which are shaped by linguistic constructions (see also Lascaratou and Marmaridou, 2005).

The view that the metaphorical understanding of pain is both reflected in and motivated by linguistic structure was further reinforced when the various conceptualisations of *ponos* were examined and the specific-level pain metaphors were derived, by focusing on the constraints emerging from the grammatical function assigned to *ponos* in each type of construction in my new material: (a) its conceptual 'objectification' effected through its grammaticalisation as object, (b) its conceptualisation as an entity located or occurring within a bounded space, i.e. the human body, and its subsequent understanding as moving within it effected through its promotion to syntactic subject of intransitive structures, denoting motion in particular, (c) its personification by virtue of its grammatical construal as subject of transitive patterns, whereby it is essentially promoted to an agent-like participant whose action can be extended to the sufferer's self, and finally (d) its clearly causal understanding structured by its construal as a circumstance of cause.

My deliberate use of a so-called 'bottom-up' approach in this investigation was motivated by my belief that in order to comprehend the metaphorical structure of pain language, we should start by analysing the various linguistic structures spontaneously uttered by a considerable number of ordinary people. On the other hand, being aware of the advantages of merging 'bottom-up' and 'top-down' approaches, in the present study I have re-interpreted my findings in the light of the generalisations and cognitive structures suggested by Kövecses (2000).

In particular, on the basis of Talmy's force dynamic schema (1988), and along the lines of Kövecses's analysis of the conceptual structure of emotions and pain, I have tried to show that the Greek pain data provide evidence in support of the view that specific-level pain metaphors are instantiations of such a general metaphor as PAIN IS A FORCE which parallels the overarching generic-level master metaphor EMOTIONS ARE FORCES. In addition, I have argued that the majority of metaphors collected in the Greek doctor-patient data focus on the cause → force (or cause → pain) causal chain of the pain scenario, motivated by the nature of doctor-patient interaction whose basic goal is to shed light on how pain is caused and sensed rather than to identify the sufferer's external action-responses (crying, screaming, whining, etc). Extending to pain Kövecses's (2000) sense of 'embodiment' proposed for emotions, I have argued that the cognitive mechanisms (conceptual metonymies and metaphors) involved are constrained by the universal aspects of the body's physiological functioning in pain, namely, the particular types of tissue damage with their accompanying sensory effects.

Along the lines of Foolen's (1997) account of the communication of emotion and on the basis of empirical evidence emerging from the data analysis, I have argued that *ponos* nominal constructions, and in particular metaphorically motivated ones, represent an *indirect* mode of externalising pain. Assuming that it is the conceptualisation of pain rather than the painful experience which is essentially communicated through the nominal framing of pain, I have claimed that, for the most part, *ponos* configurations have a stronger descriptive rather than expressive character.

Moreover, the ultimate goal of doctor-patient interaction being to bring pain under the interlocutors' control so as to eliminate it, pain must first be fully identified and explicitly described, as the analysis of the pain related dialogues suggests. My data demonstrate that this identification and description of pain is better achieved once the unpleasant sensation is metaphorically perceived as an objectified entity. That the discursively motivated objectification of pain and its subsequent personification are then discoursally fully exploited by patients and medical experts is also supported by the present analysis.

Evidence in support of this view comes from an observation first made when exploring the initial subset of doctor-patient dialogues and reconfirmed by the data in my extensive corpus: while the holistic expression of pain through the verb *ponao* is typically preferred by patients when they first present their condition, *ponos* nominal expressions of pain are usually elicited by doctors, with a view to obtaining detailed descriptions of pain. In addition, *ponos* nominal constructions are also spontaneously employed by the patients themselves in their attempt to provide explicit accounts of their painful experience. Most importantly, whether elicited by doctors or spontaneously used by patients, *ponos* metaphorical configurations are systematically resorted to after the patient's initial avowal of his pain expressed by means of a *ponao* holistic configuration.

Consider the following extract from a doctor-patient dialogue, where the patient initiates his interlocutor into his painful condition by uttering the verb form *ponao* construed as an intransitive process. In response to the doctor's question about the location of his pain, the sufferer proceeds to make an explicit description and presents PAIN AS A MOVING ENTITY that *spreads* in his body. This objectification of *ponos* finally leads to its personification as AN AGENT *setting on* the sufferer's self and alternately *squeezing* him and *letting go of* him:

(78) P: *poli, poli, para poli ponao.*
a-lot a-lot very much hurt-PRS:1SG
'*A lot, a lot, I hurt very much.*'

D: pu?
where
'Where?'

P: eδo aristera… eδo ke eδo sto poδi mu etsi… etsi *aplonete o ponos* ke meta *me xtipai* eδo sto xeri.
here on-the-left here and here in-the leg-ACC my like-this like-this spread-PRS:3SG the pain-NOM and then I-ACC strike-PRS:3SG here in-the arm-ACC
'Here on the left… here and here in my leg like this… *the pain spreads* like this and then *it strikes me* here in the arm.'

D: ne.
yes
'Yes.'

P: ala *enas ponos* etsi… *ton δexete o oryanismos tu anθropu*? *sfingi* ki *amolai, sfingi* ki *amolai.*
but a pain-NOM like-this it-ACC accept-PRS:3SG the organism-NOM the man-GEN squeeze-PRS:3SG and let-go-PRS:3SG squeeze-PRS:3SG and let-go-PRS:3SG
'But *a pain* like this… *can a man's organism take it*? *It squeezes* and *lets go, it squeezes* and *lets go*.'

To conclude, the suggestion that "such doctor-patient practices constitute the discursive, and perhaps the most significant, justification for the objectification metaphor" (Lascaratou and Marmaridou, 2005: 246) gains further support in the present study. The same discursive motivation may equally be invoked as a justification for the personification of PAIN AS A MALEVOLENT AGGRESSOR, AN IMPRISONING ENEMY, and A TORTURER. In other words, since pain is not the only domain of human experience which is treated in personification terms but rather the personification of causes of events is also quite commonly observed (see Jackendoff and Aaron, 1991), its motivation must be sought in the needs and practices which are specifically characteristic of doctor-patient discourse. Most importantly, it is suggested that, in addition to being constrained by the body's physiological functioning in pain, the metaphorical representation of the variable intensity and qualities of pain in terms of a range of metonymically derived (physical) causes (i.e. a variety of instruments or forces, e.g. SHARP OBJECT, STING, NEEDLE, KNIFE, and PHYSICAL FORCE) is also discoursally motivated and exploited. Thus, assuming that certain types of pain can be anchored to recurrent types of experience which have unambiguous observable causes (e.g. a cut with a sharp knife, piercing with a needle, a bee sting, a blow with a fist), it may be suggested that such public 'anchors' for types of pain are used to structure pain metaphorically with a view to communicating the various types of the sensation in publicly shared, i.e. 'recognisable', terms.

CHAPTER 9

Conclusions

In what follows, the main conclusions of this study are presented. One of its major contributions is that, though it is based on data from one language, i.e. Greek, its most important aspects could certainly serve to make up a framework for the cross-linguistic study of the construal of pain. Such aspects are, for example:

- the collection of a corpus of naturally-occurring dialogues between a considerable number of pain-suffering individuals and health care professionals, to form the empirical basis of a linguistic analysis of pain in everyday life and, hence, the selection of a so-called 'bottom-up' approach to the study of pain language;
- the analysis of both the lexico-grammatical construal and the metaphorical conceptualisation of physical pain in ordinary language;
- the understanding of the degree of involvement of the sufferer's self in the painful experience as a fundamental factor determining the character of its linguistic framing;
- the interpretation of the observed prevalence of the verbal framing of pain in Greek in terms of an understanding of verb forms, and in particular of intransitive ones (e.g. first-person *ponao* avowals and third-person *ponai* utterances), as the most intense construal of the experiencer's active involvement in the painful sensation, a more direct form of voicing automatic reactions: its predominantly intransitive quality as a special grammatical property contributing to the construal of pain as an inner activity or a self-induced processual event;
- the claim that the metaphorical conceptualisations of pain observed in *ponos* nominal constructions are constrained by the grammaticalisation of *ponos* as object or subject of (in)transitive structures, as part of the more general claim expressed in cognitive semantic terms, namely, that conceptualisations of everyday experience are shaped by linguistic structure, i.e. by language-specific syntactico-semantic constraints, while the linguistic realisation of metaphors and the selection of particular lexical frames are motivated by image schematic conceptual structure;

- the application of the force dynamic schema to the metaphorical representations of pain and the claim that specific-level pain metaphors are instantiations of the generic-level metaphor PAIN IS A FORCE;
- the analysis of specific-level pain metaphors as being constrained by the universal functioning of the human body in pain (the particular types of actual or potential tissue damage and their accompanying sensory effects); and
- the schematic representation of the dual function of pain along an expressive-descriptive axis in the proposed integrating continuum of pain manifestations.

1. The frequency counts applied to the collected pain patterns in the corpus of doctor-patient dialogues on which this study is based have provided me with the necessary empirical evidence in support of the characterisation of the lexico-grammatical construal of pain in Greek initially put forward in Lascaratou and Hatzidaki (2002). Hence, on the basis of the validation offered by the relevant frequency counts, I can confidently maintain that in everyday encounters Greek construes this domain of human experience as primarily verbal denoting a process (60.01%), secondarily nominal denoting a participant (38.41%), and only marginally adjectival denoting a quality (1.58%). I have, thus, been able to provide an answer to the '*what* kind' question addressed by Halliday (1998: 11) concerning the nature of the construal of this domain of human experience, in a language other than English.

2. My assumption that it is the degree of involvement of the sufferer's self in the painful experience which greatly determines the character of its lexico-grammatical construal – with the process expressing it *par excellence*, the participant following, and quality and circumstance featuring at the other end – essentially converges with Wierzbicka's (1992) cross-linguistic and cross-cultural analysis of the construction of emotions. Thus, according to Wierzbicka, the framing of emotions as verbs in a given language reflects their conceptualisation as inner activities, while their realisation as adjectives is associated with their conceptualisation as passive states brought about by external and/or past causes.

In particular, my understanding of verbal pain avowals in Greek as utterances which intensely bring out the experiencer's active involvement in the pain process finds theoretical ground in Wierzbicka's interpretation of the verbal pattern in construction of emotions as their most active, dynamic, and public linguistic expression. I suggest, therefore, that it is precisely because verb constructions offer a more direct and social processual framing of pain that they are typically preferred in Greek against the more neutral and passive adjectival frames. Consequently, with respect to the communication of pain, Greek functions very much like Russian and unlike English in the construction of emotions.

3. The following eight configurations of pain as process were observed in both patients' and doctors' data in the same descending order of frequency: (1) *ponao / ponas (eδo)* 'I hurt / I'm hurting (here)' 'do you hurt / are you hurting (here)?' (46.82%), (2) *ponai (eδo)* 'it hurts / it's hurting (here)' (19.66%), (3) *to xeri mu (mu) ponai* 'my arm hurts / my arm's hurting (in me)' (14.75%), (4) *me ponai (eδo)* 'it hurts me / it's hurting me (here)' (6.59%), (5) *to xeri mu me ponai* 'my arm's hurting me' (6.03%), (6) *afto ponai* 'that hurts' (2.90%), (7) *(afto) me ponai* 'that's hurting me' (2.35%), (8) *me ponas / se ponao*? 'you're hurting me' / 'am I hurting you?' (0.90%).

By far the most frequent of these eight structures is the intransitive-personal *ponao / ponas (eδo)* 'I hurt / I'm hurting (here)' / 'do you hurt / are you hurting (here)?', representing almost half of them (46.82%), while the intransitive-impersonal *ponai (eδo)* 'it hurts / it's hurting (here)', which is the second most frequently observed pattern, covers one fifth of the material (19.66%). Besides, three configurations occurred quite marginally, namely, *afto ponai* 'that hurts', *(afto) me ponai* 'that's hurting me', and *me ponas / se ponao*? 'you're hurting me' / 'am I hurting you?', amounting altogether to only 6.15%.

4. What my findings clearly indicate is that while Greek pain constructions are consistently, on the one hand, intransitive and, on the other, personal, their intransitive nature is more prevalent.

The principally intransitive quality of pain as process in Greek can be associated with the significance attributed by Wierzbicka (1992) to the largely intransitive nature of Russian verbs in framing emotions as a special grammatical property whereby emotions are understood as inner activities and active, self-induced, processual events.

In addition, I propose that the observed intransitive dimension in the processual construal of pain in Greek is also highlighted by the assumed superiority of intransitive verbs over transitives, as presented in a number of psycholinguistic and neurolinguistic studies (e.g. De Bleser and Kauschke, 2003, among others). To be more specific, it is suggested that there is a clear tendency among children and aphasic adults to prefer intransitive rather than transitive verbs, which can be accounted for in terms of their simpler, more accessible argument structure properties.

Drawing on this psycholinguistic claim and extending it to the construal of pain, I propose that intransitive pain constructions, and in particular first-person *ponao* avowals and third-person *ponai* utterances, are statistically predominant by virtue of their ability to function as an essentially 'simpler', a more direct form of voicing a reaction, compared to patterns configuring pain as a multi-argument process. This is further reinforced by the fact that in Greek many more vital biological and mental processes are mostly intransitively construed, e.g. *pinao* 'I'm hungry', *δipsao* 'I'm thirsty', *nistazo* 'I feel sleepy', *fovame* 'I'm afraid' and *peθeno* 'I die' / 'I'm dying'.

5. With respect to the very high frequency of first-person *ponao* 'I hurt' / 'I'm hurting' pain constructions, the exploration of the doctor-patient dialogues indicates that they often have an exclamatory function, hence, they approximate to interjections, with which they were found to co-occur or alternate quite frequently. In addition to voicing 'cries of complaint', such patterns also represent the principal formal means whereby the patient introduces himself as a suffering self, thus paving the way for the subsequent description of pain in terms of its variable properties.

In order to interpret the intensity of the construal of pain involved in *ponao* avowals, both their experiential grammar and the textual component of grammar must be appealed to. Hence, not only do these *ponao* construals encode the pain experience very vividly by bringing out its processual dimension, but in terms of textual grammar, they also create a holistic thematic perspective for the presentation of the painful sensation, given that the sufferer's self is 'incorporated' in the process *via* the verb suffix. (See also (8) below.)

6. Like intransitive-personal *ponao* avowals, intransitive-impersonal *ponai* utterances in patients' speech are primarily interpreted as "replacing the primitive cry" in Wittgenstein's (1953/1989) sense. As in the case of *ponao*, my claim about the expressive function of *ponai* is corroborated by its frequent co-occurrence with typical pain exclamations observed in the data.

The high frequency of *ponai* in the sense of 'it's hurting' can be accounted for in terms of the dynamic and actional processual construal of pain it provides, by virtue of its understanding as consisting essentially of the process only, on the analogy of clauses representing meteorological processes. Hence, through the intransitive-impersonal *ponai*, the pain experience may be symbolised as a physical phenomenon (unexpectedly) overwhelming the sufferer, much like a sudden rain or snowfall (cf. *vrexi* 'it's raining', *xionizi* 'it's snowing').

7. The various types of 'figure' into which pain as process enters in the constructions observed in the material of the present study are figures of 'doing and happening', 'sensing' or 'being'.

There are three clear cases of 'doing something to someone or something', that is, three cases of two-participant processes. What is 'done' is pain, which is induced to the person, the sufferer, (a) by an object or event, i.e. a non-conscious entity, as in one of the two patterns observed in my Greek data with no corresponding English expressions in Halliday's paradigm, namely, *afto me ponai*, 'that's hurting me', (b) by another person, usually non-volitionally, e.g. *me ponas* 'you're hurting me', and (c) by a part of the person's body, e.g. *to xeri mu me ponai*, 'my arm's hurting me'. 'Doing' merges with 'sensing' in all these cases and, in particular, in (c) where the entity causing the pain (the body part) and the person undergoing the pain make up a single entity, i.e. the sufferer.

Moreover, pain may be seen as 'happening' rather than clearly 'being done' either to a conscious entity, i.e. the sufferer, or a part of a person's body in the intransitive patterns *ponao* 'I'm hurting', and *to xeri mu ponai* 'my arm's hurting', respectively. In these cases, where current infliction of pain is expressed, 'happening' merges with 'being'. Most importantly, in the impersonal *ponai* 'it's hurting', pain takes on the further sense of 'occurring', like a meteorological process, without any reference to a particular body part as an indication of its location, which is, therefore, understood as an impersonal, i.e. abstract, setting. When *ponai*, however, corresponds to *it hurts* and is interpreted as expressing a chronic state of pain, i.e. a state of being, it acquires the further sense of 'existing'.

Pain can also appear in the form of a process essentially representing a quality attributed either to the sufferer, as in *ponao* 'I hurt', or to a part of his body, as in *to xeri mu ponai* 'my arm hurts'. Furthermore, pain, or rather the ability to cause pain, may be ascribed as an attribute to an external agent, e.g. an object or process unintentionally or accidentally bringing about an unpleasant sensation, as in *afti i eksetasi ponai* 'this test hurts / is painful'. Finally, in *me ponai* 'it hurts me' / 'it's hurting me', the second Greek pattern observed in the dialogues with no corresponding English expression featuring in Halliday's paradigm, pain enters in a figure of sensing, where the person suffers as a result of an impersonal, non-specific, unidentified cause.

The Greek data confirm Halliday's (1998: 27–28) comment that "speakers explore this highly complex domain of human experience by mapping it into figures of more or less every possible type", all of which retain, as it were, "an affiliation with what Matthiessen (1993) calls the 'conscious centre'."

8. With respect to the way the locus of pain is understood in the various configurations of pain as process, we observe that in the great majority (56.66%) of all collected constructions it is the suffering person rather than a body part which is seen as "the locus where [pain] is actualized" (Halliday 1998: 26), *ponao* 'I hurt' / 'I'm hurting' patterns covering 82.63% of such representations. My claim that in Greek pain is primarily configured as dwelling in the sufferer's self as a whole emerges chiefly from the intensity with which intransitive *ponao* avowals reflect the involvement of the self in the subjective, private experience of pain, which, I maintain, brings about the statistical prevalence of such patterns.

The sufferer's grammaticalisation as subject, 'incorporated' in the verb form *via* its suffix, allows me to relate my understanding of the vividness with which the sufferer's self and his involvement are reflected in *ponao* configurations to Kripke's

(1982: 145) interpretation of Wittgenstein's grammatical representation of the self: "In the *Investigations*, the special character of the self [...] is thought of as deriving from a 'grammatical' peculiarity of the first-person pronoun, not from any special metaphysical mystery." Thus, I assume that this 'grammatical peculiarity' of the first-person pronoun can also be extended to the first-person ending of Greek verbs. Hence, I suggest that *ponao* utterances can often be understood as directly expressing the pain experience of the suffering self, very much like a cry does.

Consequently, the data analysis of my extensive corpus reinforces the claim put forward in Lascaratou and Hatzidaki (2002: 71) that in Greek "it is primarily the self which is configured as the setting of the painful condition" and that "pain is understood as residing in the sufferer's self as a whole rather than in just some part of it."

9. The 'actualisation' of pain in the sufferer's body as a whole takes up several forms. Thus, in first-person *ponao* avowals, where the suffering person is linguistically realised through the verb suffix, he is construed as experiencing pain holistically. The sufferer is assigned the functions of Carrier, Actor, or Behaver, or he may function as a kind of Setting where pain is understood to dwell or occur. On the other hand, in *me ponas* / *se ponao*? 'you're hurting me' / 'am I hurting you?' and *afto me ponai* 'that's hurting me', the person is conceived as the Goal of the painful process, while in the impersonal *me ponai* 'it hurts me' / 'it's hurting me' the sufferer is represented as the Senser of pain.

In about one fifth of the collected patterns (19.66%) pain appears as residing in an impersonal, non-specific, abstract, virtual Setting. This is the case of the intransitive impersonal *ponai* 'it hurts' / 'it's hurting', where neither the sufferer nor any body part is linguistically realised. I suggest that impersonal *ponai* structures could also be interpreted as expressing the involvement of the sufferer's self and his related feelings of confinement and entrapment, as these feelings may often deprive him of the ability to describe his pain explicitly in terms of a tangible and concrete setting.

Finally, in only one more fifth of the data (20.78%) where pain is construed as a process, is the locus of pain identified with a part of the sufferer's body rather than with the sufferer's self configured holistically. More specifically, in *to xeri mu ponai* 'my arm hurts / is hurting' (14.75%), the sufferer specifies the part of his body that is painful by configuring it either as the Carrier of the painful sensation or the Actor, i.e. the 'doer of the deed', or as a kind of Setting where pain simply occurs or exists. Moreover, in *to xeri mu me ponai* 'my arm's hurting me' (6.03%), the body part – in the form of a distinct clause element – participates in a material process as an external Agent, hence explicitly identifying the locus of the painful experience.

10. The lexico-grammatical analysis of pain as thing, linguistically realised by *ponos* nominal expressions, in terms of the seven pain features identified by Halliday (1998) and exemplified with naturally-occurring Greek data, has confirmed the cross-linguistic applicability and validity of these properties as dimensions along which the painful sensation may be made an 'object' of description, measurement and assessment.

These grammatically construed semantic properties are: *ponos* (a) may be construed as a bounded or an unbounded entity, (b) is a possession (c) has temporal location and extent, (d) has accompanying conditions, (e) has variable location within the body, (f) varies in intensity, and (g) manifests variable qualities. However, only the diverse qualities of pain are actually criterial for its categorisation and qualification, i.e. are exclusively related to this sensation, the other attributes expressing general features of many other types of phenomena, though they also significantly contribute to the identification and assessment of this domain of human experience.

Here is a brief summary of the most significant aspects of these features: (a) The understanding of *ponos* as either a bounded or an unbounded entity plays a crucial part in the interpretation of constructions where it is grammaticalised as the object of the verbs *exo* 'have', *esθanome* 'feel', and *njoθo* 'feel' (e.g. *otan exo ton ponokefalo, δen pino* 'when I have the headache, I don't drink', *njoθis eki pono*? 'do you feel pain there?') (see also (13) below); (b) Pain as thing is an undesired possession that the sufferer may acquire, receive, or own (e.g. *aftus tus ponus tus ksanaixa* 'I've had these pains again'), and which, in any case, he struggles hard to free himself from, to 'lose'; (c) Besides their adverbial construal, the temporal characteristics of pain may also be metaphorically expressed as a quality in the form of an adjective (e.g. *sinexis* 'continuous', *δiarkis* 'constant', *monimos* 'permanent', *xronios* 'chronic'), or (d) they may additionally be identified in terms of accompanying conditions, grammatically construed as a temporal nexus (e.g. *o ponos arxizi otan sikoθo* 'the pain starts when I stand up); (e) In addition to being specified by means of an adverbial (e.g. *eδo mesa* 'in here', *eki* 'there') or an adjective (e.g. *topikos* 'local', *endopizmenos* 'localised') or a compound noun indicating the painful body part (e.g. *ponokefalos* 'headache'), the variable location of pain within the body is also quite commonly depicted as some kind of 'path' through which pain 'travels' in the sufferer's body. Hence, the basic metaphorical understanding of *ponos* as a moving entity emerges, setting the scene for its personification (see (13) below); (f) and (g) Degree of intensity and quality of pain are often not easily distinguishable from each other. Hence, semantic features related to both intensity and quality frequently appear amalgamated in the form of adjectives, e.g. *ylikos* 'sweet', and *oksis* 'sharp', while some pain descriptors can even be interpreted as expressing more than one qualitative properties, e.g. *vaθis* 'deep'. Moreover, adjectives are also used for the grammatical representation of mere pain intensity (e.g. *δinatos ponos* 'strong pain', *aforiti poni* 'unbearable pains'), its measurement being one of the most difficult aspects of pain assessment.

The Greek version of the McGill Pain Questionnaire in its short form (GR-SFMPQ) has served as a technical basis for my analysis of the qualitative differences of pain properties and the categorisation of the descriptors collected in the dialogues. It is noteworthy that the majority of sensory pain qualities featuring in the GR-SFMPQ are linguistically represented by means of metaphorically structured adjectives or adjectival participles both in the original English terms and their Greek translation equivalents.

The metaphorical structuring of Greek sensory pain descriptors was confirmed by the data analysis, where it was observed that, as in English, they are figures of speech whereby, by virtue of a particular pain quality, the sensation is likened to the mode of (or the instrument / means used in) an unpleasant, harmful, or aggressive action which may cause injury or pain, and that an observable, 'natural' and physical process is implicated. Thus, on the basis of the general metonymic relationship INSTRUMENT / MEANS FOR ACTION / EVENT, a range of (physical) causes are metonymically derived which are subsequently applied for the metaphorical representation of the various sensory qualities of pain, in terms of sensory pain descriptors. What is more, in the doctor-patient dialogues, metaphorical descriptors are not only spontaneously produced by the patient, they are also quite commonly elicited by means of explicit clues supplied by the health professional, who may thus provide the patient with the conceptual source domain from which he can structure his pain experience.

That pain is a multifaceted domain of everyday life is reflected in the difficulty I experienced in my attempt to map the sensory pain descriptors and the intensity terms observed in the authentic dialogues onto those of such a reliable and valid assessment tool as the GR-SFMPQ. I suggest that this is an indication that, despite their diversity and multitude, our conventional linguistic labels whereby pain is classified into categories are ultimately exceeded by our actual pain experiences.

11. In its construal as thing, pain, i.e. *ponos*, is understood as entering directly as a 'participant' into three of Halliday's four primary types of figure, namely, 'doing', 'sensing', and 'being and having', while no case of 'saying' corresponding structurally to the original English pattern *the pain suggests that*… was observed.

'Doing something to someone' is represented by construction *afto mu δini / ferni / prokali ponokefalo* 'that's giving / bringing / causing me a headache', realised as a three-participant process, with *ponos* 'pain' understood as what is 'done' (Goal) rather than the 'doer' and induced to the sufferer by a non-conscious entity, i.e. an object or an event. Moreover, *ponos* participates in the figure of 'sensing' represented by *njoθis eki pono*? 'do you feel any pain there?', as that which is perceived (Phenomenon). Pain may also enter into a figure of 'being' either (a) as a thing (Carrier) described in terms of an attribute, e.g. *o ponos mu ine avastaxtos ti nixta* 'my pain is intolerable at night', or (b) as a thing (Identified) measured by means of a Token (Identifier), or (c) as a thing that simply exists (Existent), exemplified by the additional two Greek cases observed in my material, namely, *to 10 ine o aforitos ponos* 'score 10 is / represents the excruciating pain' and *ine enas ponos eδo* 'there is (a) pain here' (where 'being' merges with 'existing'), respectively. Finally, in cases of 'having', pain may be conceived as a possession (possessed Attribute), either owned by the sufferer, e.g. *exo pono sti mesi* 'I've got (a) pain in the / my low back', or granted / caused to the sufferer, e.g. *afto mu δini / ferni / prokali ponokefalo* 'that gives / brings / causes me a headache'.

12. In the cognitive semantic account of the metaphorical conceptualisation of pain in Greek on the basis of the set of *ponos* nominal constructions observed in the corpus, I have essentially chosen to follow a so-called 'bottom-up' approach. My choice is a conscious and deliberate one: I believe that, to gain an understanding of the metaphorical structure of pain language, it is indispensable to proceed by first examining the actual linguistic constructions spontaneously uttered by different ordinary people, either at the time they experience the painful sensation or when they attempt to describe it. This does not mean, however, that I do not appreciate the advantages of a 'top-down' approach, whereby cognitive scholars, mostly relying on selective evidence provided by highly conventionalised metaphorical linguistic expressions, aim at proposing generalisations and underlying global cognitive structures that may interpret the linguistic data. On the contrary, it is my belief that the investigation of the conceptual structure of pain can only benefit from the 'merging' of 'bottom-up' and 'top-down' approaches. Hence, I have attempted to complement my approach by re-interpreting my findings in the light of Kövecses's (2000) 'top-down' analysis of metaphor in emotion and its application to the investigation of the conceptual structure of pain (Kövecses, forth.).

13. The revised cognitive semantic analysis of *ponos* nominal constructions in the present study, has confirmed the validity of the central claim originally expressed in Lascaratou and Marmaridou (2005), namely, that these patterns are systematically motivated by both language-specific syntactico-semantic constraints and conceptual metaphors.

The close relation holding between the metaphorical understanding of pain and its linguistic realisations was once more brought to light when I looked into the various conceptualisations of *ponos*, with respect to the grammatical function it is assigned, in each type of structure observed in the material of this study.

Thus, as the grammatical object of the possessive *exo*, *ponos* is construed as an objectified possessed entity, hence becoming a referent in discourse independent of the sufferer, e.g. *δen ton ixa afton ton pono* 'I didn't have this pain'. This objectification, both grammatical and conceptual, facilitates doctors and patients in their attempts to identify, describe, and measure pain.

Moreover, once *ponos* has gained conceptual distance from the sufferer, which is iconically reflected in the relevant structures, it may make one more step further and be grammaticalised as the subject of intransitive verbs. In such processes, *ponos* is 'promoted' to the initiator or Actor and may be construed as an event bounded in time, e.g. *mu ixe perasi o ponos ke meta mu ksanarxise pali* 'the pain had passed (had left me) and then it started again', or a force of variable quality fluctuating in intensity, e.g. *i poni arxisan na δinamonun* 'the pains started to get stronger'. What is more, the grammaticalisation of *ponos* as subject of motion verbs and, hence, its construal as initiator of its own movement leads to its understanding as a self-willed animate entity moving within a bounded space, i.e. the human body, e.g. *erxete o ponos, fevji, ksanarxete* 'the pain comes and goes, comes back again'.

Profiled as an animate entity, *ponos* is further grammaticalised as subject in transitive processes of 'doing something to someone else', thus acquiring the feature of agentivity, by virtue of which it is personified. My additional data lend support to the earlier observation that the grammaticalisation of *ponos* as subject of transitive verbs motivates a number of very closely related conceptualisations in which the feature of animacy involved in the ontological metaphor of personification is fully exploited. For example, *ponos* is configured as a malevolent aggressor setting on the sufferer, e.g. *apotoma mja mera m' epjase enas ponos*, 'suddenly one day a pain set on me', a ruthless torturer, e.g. *me pniji… me sfingi… me travai* 'it strangles me… it squeezes me… it pulls me', and, ultimately, as an immobilising and imprisoning enemy, e.g. *δe m' afini na sikoθo*, 'it (the pain) does not let me stand up'. Eventually, *ponos* may resume its initial grammatical status of object, not any more as a possessed entity, however, but as the entity to be confronted and, hopefully, defeated by the patient, e.g. *exo θesi ipo elenxo tus ponus* 'I have set the pains under control'. Finally, construed as a circumstance of cause, *ponos* is understood in clearly causal terms, e.g. *lipoθimisa / ksipnao apo ton pono / tus ponus* 'I fainted / wake up from the pain(s)', *peθeno stus ponus*, 'I die from the pains'.

14. Following up Lascaratou and Marmaridou (2005), Talmy's (1988) force dynamic schema was invoked to interpret those conceptualisations of pain emerging from two-participant clauses where *ponos* is grammaticalised as an agentive subject whose action is extended to, or directed at, the (sufferer's) self. Assuming that this schema – in which two forces are represented as interacting – best captures aspects of agentivity and causativity, the (sufferer's) self was mapped onto the Ago-

nist, i.e. the contestant, confronted with a counteracting force, namely, (the cause of) his pain, mapped onto the Antagonist, i.e. his opponent.

However, the analysis of the new material on which the present study is based called for a revision of the initial account. In revising the earlier account, I have also systematically associated and contrasted my proposed amended version to Kövecses (2000 and forth.). In particular, in the light of Kövecses's analysis, I have attempted to show that my doctor-patient data provide empirical evidence from a language other than English in support of the view that specific-level pain metaphors are instantiations of such a general metaphor as PAIN IS A FORCE which parallels the metaphor EMOTIONS ARE FORCES proposed by Kövecses as an overarching generic-level master metaphor in emotion.

15. Extending to pain the specific and limited sense of 'embodiment' that Kövecses (2000) proposes for emotions, I have argued that the cognitive mechanisms (conceptual metonymies and metaphors) underlying the specific-level Greek pain metaphors are motivated, i.e. they are constrained by, the universal aspects of human physiology in pain. Hence, on the basis of the evidence provided by the Greek doctor-patient data, I have claimed that the conceptualisations of pain can only emerge within the constraints imposed by the particular types of (actual or potential) tissue damage and their accompanying sensory effects associated with the experience of pain, i.e. they cannot contradict the universal aspects of the functioning of the human body in pain.

16. In this study I have endorsed the view that the various aspects of the metaphorical understanding of pain emerging from the analysis of my authentic data have 'real world' motivation, i.e. are experientially grounded. Thus for example, every person's experience that the sensation of pain with its distressing effects typically appears unexpectedly, often impeding one's activity or even threatening one's existence, constitutes the experiential basis for the metaphorical understanding of *ponos* as an alien invader, a ruthless torturer and, ultimately, a confining and paralysing enemy.

17. On the basis of new empirical evidence derived from the extensive corpus, but without engaging in any systematic treatment of discourse-pragmatic factors, I have been able to suggest more convincingly, I believe, that, in addition to being linguistically motivated, *ponos* metaphorical construals whereby pain is objectified are also motivated, exploited and sustained by doctor-patient discourse practices. In particular, the analysis of the pain-related dialogues suggests that the metaphorical conceptualisation of pain as an objectified entity and its subsequent personification is motivated by the ultimate goal of doctor-patient interaction, which is to fully identify and explicitly describe the unpleasant sensation so as to bring it

under the interlocutors' control and eventually eliminate it. What is more, I have argued that it is the vital necessity to reach an understanding of how pain is caused and sensed, rather than how the patient externalises it, which motivates the focus taken by the majority of the collected Greek pain metaphors on the causes of the painful experience, rather than on the patient's related action-responses (weeping, screaming, groaning, etc). In addition, I have suggested that the metaphorical representation of the various qualities and degrees of pain in terms of a variety of instruments or forces, e.g. STING, NEEDLE, SHARP OBJECT / KNIFE, and PHYSICAL FORCE (i.e. a range of metonymically derived (physical) causes) is not only constrained by the functioning of the human body in pain, but it is also discoursally motivated and exploited. Thus, it may be suggested that certain types of experience unambiguously causing a variety of painful sensations, such as a bee sting, piercing with a needle, a cut with a sharp knife, a blow with a fist, etc., are used to structure pain metaphorically with a view to communicating the various types of the sensation in publicly shared, i.e. 'recognisable' terms, by virtue of being publicly observable and recurrent.

18. Mapping my proposed analysis of the function of pain utterances in terms of a continuum of (verbal and non-verbal) pain manifestations onto Foolen's (1997) account of the communication of emotion has allowed me to propose that specific forms of the processual construal of pain in Greek can sometimes be identified with a potential direct linguistic expression of pain, as the corpus data suggest.

In particular, I have claimed that intransitive (either first-person *ponao* 'I hurt' / 'I'm hurting' or impersonal third-person *ponai* 'it hurts' / 'it's hurting') pain avowals, especially when used on their own, often have an exclamatory function. Therefore, I suggest that these patterns are used by the sufferer primarily to express – rather than describe – his painful sensation. What is more, the observation that *ponao* / *ponai* utterances quite frequently co-occur or alternate with pain exclamations in the corpus (such as *axa!* / *ax!* / *a!* / *u!* / *ox!* / *oxu!* 'ah!' / 'oh!' / 'ouch!') lends further support to the graphic representation of such instances of the specific verb forms in positions next to interjections, since the latter are assumed to be the linguistic signs located most closely to the proposed expressive pole of pain behaviour (which comprises automatic non-linguistic pain reactions, i.e. cries / groans / screams), that is one of the two extreme ends of the continuum.

To complete the schematic representation of the processual framing of pain in a manner that will bring out the assumed gradience of its expressive function, I propose the following symbolic arrangement of the collected patterns as we move along the expressive-descriptive axis of the continuum: *ponao* (*eδo*) 'I hurt / I'm hurting (here)' > *ponai* (*eδo*) 'it hurts / it's hurting (here)' > *me ponai* (*eδo*) 'it hurts me / it's hurting me (here)' > *to xeri mu* (*mu*) *ponai* 'my arm hurts / my arm's hurting (in me)' > *to xeri mu me ponai* 'my arm's hurting me' > *afto ponai* 'that hurts' > (*afto*) *me ponai* 'that's hurting me' > *me ponas* / *se ponao*? 'you're hurting me' / 'am I hurting you?'.

19. As for *ponos* constructions, I have assumed that they constitute an indirect channel of externalising pain, whereby the conceptualisation of pain precedes its verbalisation. In particular, I have presented empirical evidence in support of my claim that what is communicated when pain is linguistically realised by means of explicit, metaphorically motivated, *ponos* constructions is the conceptualisation of pain rather than the painful experience itself.

What is more, I have provided further linguistic, cognitive, and discursive justification for the claim that metaphorically structured *ponos* configurations should be placed at the extreme pole of the proposed integrating continuum of pain manifestations representing the descriptive function of pain language (see Lascaratou and Marmaridou, 2005), just opposite the other extreme one representing automatic, primitive pain reactions. Hence, I have been able to identify the objectifying, descriptive and reportive character of such metaphorical structures more thoroughly.

Finally, on the basis of my data analysis I have argued that, on the whole, the nominal construction of pain in terms of *ponos* 'pain', featuring as a participant, has a stronger descriptive rather than expressive function, unlike its verbal framing through the various forms of the *ponao* 'I hurt' verb paradigm.

20. Finally, my data-based study of how pain, as a domain of human experience, is transformed into language in terms of its lexico-grammar in Greek, essentially converges with Wittgenstein's (1953/1989) philosophical interpretation of the dual function of pain language as primarily an expression of this sensation, also potentially entailing a description. Moreover, the Greek data have shown that there are 'transitions' between a cry of complaint and a description of a state of mind, i.e. that the distinction between expression and description cannot always be sharply drawn.

To conclude, having attempted to provide an answer concerning the function of pain language, I cannot avoid speculating as to whether the possibility of expressing or describing pain through language essentially refutes the subjective, private character of pain. Thus, despite the variety of the linguistic means observed in doctor-patient dialogues, whereby the sufferer attempts to communicate pain in socially shared terms, I cannot but wonder with Schweizer (1995: 211) whether suffering ultimately remains *unheard* and *speechless*. Could one eliminate the possibility that pain remains an essentially unsharable and profoundly solitary confining experience, one that brings about an "absolute split between one's sense of one's own reality and the reality of other persons", as Elaine Scarry (1985: 4) argues?

Indeed, is there anyone who has not at some point felt in tune with Scarry who suggests that,

> for the person in pain, so incontestably and unnegotiably present is it that "having pain" may come to be thought of as the most vibrant example of what it is to "have certainty," while for the other person it is so elusive that "hearing about pain" may exist as the primary model of what it is "to have doubt." Thus pain comes unsharably into our midst as at once that which cannot be denied and that which cannot be confirmed.

References

Aldrich, Sarah and Eccleston, Chris. 2000. "Making sense of everyday pain". *Social Science and Medicine* 50: 1631–1641.

Antonopoulou, Eleni. 1987. "Prototype Theory and the Meaning of Verbs, with Special Reference to Modern Greek Verbs of Motion." Unpublished Ph.D. thesis, University of London.

Ashburn, Michael A. and Rice, Linda J. 1998. *The Management of Pain*. Philadelphia: Churchill Livingstone.

Athanasiadou, Angeliki and Tabakowska, Elzbieta. (eds). 1998. *Speaking of Emotions: Conceptualization and Expression*. Berlin: Mouton de Gruyter.

Bacchini, Simone. forth. "'This is my pain': Agency and individuality in the experience of an Italian woman with chronic illness. A linguistic approach." In *Reconstructing Pain and Joy: Linguistic, Literary, and Cultural Perspectives*, Chryssoula Lascaratou, Anna Despotopoulou and Elly Ifantidou (eds), Newcastle, UK: Cambridge Scholars Publishing.

Bamberg, Michael. 1997. "Emotion talk(s): The role of perspective in the construction of emotions." In *The Language of Emotions*, Susanne Niemeier and René Dirven (eds), 209–225. Amsterdam: John Benjamins.

Baszanger, Isabelle. 1992. "Deciphering chronic pain." *Sociology of Health and Illness* 14 (2): 181–215.

Biber, Douglas. 1993. "Representativeness in corpus design." *Literary and Linguistic Computing* 8 (4): 243–257.

Biber, Douglas, Conrad, Susan and Reppen, Randi. 1998. *Corpus Linguistics. Investigating Language Structure and Use*. Cambridge: Cambridge University Press.

Bloom, Lois. 1993a. *The Transition from Infancy to Language: Acquiring the Power of Expression*. Cambridge: Cambridge University Press.

Bloom, Lois. 1993b. "Language and the powers of expression." In *Language and Communication: Comparative Perspectives*, Herbert Roitblat et al. (eds), 95–113. Hillsdale, N.J.: Lawrence Erlbaum.

Borsook, David, LeBel, Alyssa A. and McPeek, Bucknam. 1998. *Εγχειρίδιο Αντιμετώπισης του Πόνου του Massachusetts General Hospital* [Massachusetts General Hospital Handbook of Pain Management]. Translated by Sonia Kamvisi-Dea. Athens: Litsas.

Brugman, Claudia. 1988. "The Syntax and Semantics of HAVE and its Complements." Ph.D. thesis, University of California, Berkeley.

Cameron, Lynne and Deignan, Alice. 2003. "Combining large and small corpora to investigate tuning devices around metaphor in spoken discourse." *Metaphor and Symbol* 18 (3): 149–160.

Crowdy, Steve. 1993. "Spoken corpus design." *Literary and Linguistic Computing* 8 (4): 159–265.

Damasio, Antonio R. 1999. *The Feeling of What Happens*. New York: Harcourt Brace and Company.

Davidoff, Jules and Masterson, Jackie. 1995. "The development of picture naming: Differences between verbs and nouns." *Journal of Neurolinguistics* 9: 69–83.

De Beaugrande, Robert. 2001. "Large corpora, small corpora, and the learning of 'language'." In *Small Corpus Studies and ELT*, Mohsen Ghadessy, Alex Henry and Robert L. Roseberry (eds), 3–28. Amsterdam: John Benjamins.

De Bleser, Ria and Kauschke, Christina. 2003. "Acquisition and loss of nouns and verbs: Parallel or divergent patterns?" *Journal of Neurolinguistics* 16: 213–229.

Deignan, Alice. 1999a. "Corpus-based research into metaphor." In *Researching and Applying Metaphor*, Lynne Cameron and Graham Low (eds), 177–199. Cambridge: Cambridge University Press.

Deignan, Alice. 1999b. "Linguistic metaphors and collocation in nonliterary corpus data." *Metaphor and Symbol* 14 (1): 19–36.

Deignan, Alice. 2005a. "A corpus linguistic perspective on the relationship between metonymy and metaphor." *Style* 39 (1): 72–91.

Deignan, Alice. 2005b. *Metaphor and Corpus Linguistics*. Amsterdam: John Benjamins.

Del Veccio Good, Mary-Jo, Brodwin, Paul E., Good, Byron J. and Kleinman, Arthur (eds). 1992. *Pain as Human Experience: An Anthropological Perspective*. Berkeley: University of California Press.

DeSouza, Lorraine H. and Frank, Andrew O. 2000. "Subjective pain experience of people with chronic back pain." *Physiotherapy Research International* 5 (4): 207–219.

Drachman, Gaberell. 1985. "Language universals – the two approaches." In *Studia Linguistica Diachronica et Synchronica*, Ursula Pieper and Gerhard Stickel (eds), 175–201. The Hague: Mouton.

Edwards, Lindsey C. and Pearce, Shirley A. 1994. "Word completion in chronic pain: Evidence for schematic representation of pain." *Journal of Abnormal Psychology* 103 (2): 379–382.

Ekman, Paul. 1980. *The Face of Man. Expressions of Universal Emotions in a New Guinea Village*. New York: Garland.

Ekman, Paul. 1992. "An argument for basic emotions." *Cognition and Emotions* 6: 169–200.

Ekman, Paul. 1993. "Facial expression and emotion." *American Psychologist* 48 (4): 384–392.

Enfield, Nick J. and Wierzbicka, Anna. 2002. "Introduction: The body in description of emotion." *Pragmatics and Cognition* 10 (1–2): 1–25.

Enfield, Nick J. and Wierzbicka, Anna (eds). 2002. *Pragmatics and Cognition* 10 (1–2). Special issue on *The Body in Description of Emotion: Cross-Linguistic Studies*. Amsterdam: John Benjamins.

Engel, George. 1950. "Psychogenic pain and the pain-prone patient." *American Journal of Medicine* 26: 899–909.

Fabrega, Horatio Jr and Tyma, Stephen. 1976a. "Culture, language, and the shaping of illness: An illustration based on pain." *Journal of Psychosomatic Research* 20: 323–337.

Fabrega, Horatio Jr and Tyma, Stephen. 1976b. "Language and cultural influences in the description of pain." *British Journal of Psychology* 49: 349–371.

Fernandez, Ephrem and Towery, Stuart. 1996. "A parsimonious set of verbal descriptors of pain sensation derived from the McGill Pain Questionnaire." *Pain* 66: 31–37.

Foolen, Ad. 1997. "The expressive function of language: Towards a cognitive semantic approach." In *The Language of Emotions*, Susanne Niemeier and René Dirven (eds), 15–31. Amsterdam: John Benjamins.

Foucault, Michel. 1991. *The Birth of the Clinic: An Archaeology of Medical Perception*. London: Routledge.

Foucault, Michel. 1992. *The Order of Things: An Archaeology of the Human Sciences*. London: Routledge.

Freud, Sigmund. 1915a/1956. "Repression." *Collected Papers*, Vol. IV. London: The Hogarth Press.

Freud, Sigmund. 1915b/1984. "Repression." *On Metapsychology: The Theory of Psychoanalysis.* The Pelican Freud Library, Vol. 11. Middlesex: Penguin Books.

Freud, Sigmund. 1915c/1984. "The unconscious." *On Metapsychology: The Theory of Psychoanalysis.* The Pelican Freud Library, Vol. 11. Middlesex: Penguin Books.

Freud, Sigmund. 1926. "Inhibitions, symptoms and anxiety." *On Psychopathology: Inhibitions Symptoms and Anxiety and Other Works*. The Pelican Freud Library, Vol. 10. Middlesex: Penguin Books.

Fries, Peter. H. 1981/1983. "On the status of theme in English: Arguments from discourse." *Forum Linguisticum* 6 (1): 1–38. Revised version in *Micro and Macro Connexity of Texts*, Janos S. Petöfi and Emile Sözer (eds), 116–152. Hamburg: Buske.

Fries, Peter. H. 1992. "The structuring of written English text." *Language Sciences* 14 (4): 461–488.

Fries, Peter. H. 1995. "Themes, methods of development, and texts." In *On Subject and Theme: A Discourse Functional Perspective*, Ruqaiya Hasan and Peter H. Fries (eds), 317–359. Amsterdam: John Benjamins.

Gaston-Johansson, Fannie. 1984. "Pain assessment: Differences in quality and intensity of the words pain, ache, and hurt." *Pain* 20: 69–76.

Georgoudis, George, Oldham, Jacqueline A. and Watson, Paul J. 2001. "Reliability and sensitivity measures of the Greek version of the short form of the McGill Pain Questionnaire." *European Journal of Pain* 5: 109–118.

Georgoudis, George, Watson, Paul J. and Oldham, Jacqueline A. 2000. "The development and validation of a Greek version of the short-form McGill Pain Questionnaire." *European Journal of Pain* 4: 275–281.

Gergen, Kenneth J. 1991. *The Saturated Self: Dilemmas of Identity in Contemporary Life*. Basic Books.

Ghadessy, Mohsen (ed.). 1995. *Thematic Development in English Texts*. London: Pinter.

Gibbon, Daffyd, Moore, Roger, and Winski, Richard. 1998. *Spoken Language Characterisation*, Vol. 2. Berlin: Mouton de Gruyter.

Gibbs, Raymond W. 1999. "Researching metaphor." In *Researching and Applying Metaphor*, Lynne Cameron and Graham Low (eds), 29–47. Cambridge: Cambridge University Press.

Gibbs, Raymond W. 2006. *Embodiment and Cognitive Science*. Cambridge: Cambridge University Press.

Goldstein, Irwin. 2000. "Intersubjective properties by which we specify pain, pleasure, and other kinds of mental states." *Philosophy* 75: 89–104.

Greenberg, Joseph H. 1963/1966. "Some universals of grammar with particular reference to the order of meaningful elements." In *Universals of Language*, Joseph H. Greenberg (ed.), 73–113. Cambridge, Massachusetts: MIT Press.

Gustafson, Donald F. 1979. "'Pain', grammar and physicalism." In *Body, Mind and Method. Essays in Honor of Virgil C. Aldrich*, Donald F. Gustafson and Bangs L. Tapscott (eds), 149–166. Dordrecht: D. Reidel Publishing Company.

Gwyn, Richard. 1999. "Captain of my own ship: Metaphor and the discourse of chronic illness." In *Researching and Applying Metaphor*, Lynne Cameron and Graham Low (eds), 203–220. Cambridge: Cambridge University Press.

Haiman, John. 1983. "Iconic and economic motivation." *Language* 59: 781–819.

Hallberg, Lillemor R.-M. and Carlsson, Sven G. 2000. "Coping with fibromyalgia: A qualitative study." *Scandinavian Journal of Caring Sciences* 14: 29–36.

Halliday, Michael Alexander Kirkwood. 1985/1994. *An Introduction to Functional Grammar*. London and New York: Pinter.

Halliday, Michael Alexander Kirkwood. 1998. "On the grammar of pain." *Functions of Language* 5 (1): 1–32.

Harre, Rom. 1991. "The discursive production of selves." *Theory and Psychology* 1 (1): 51–63.

Hasan, Ruqaiya and Fries, Peter H. (eds). 1995. *On Subject and Theme: A Discourse Functional Perspective*. Amsterdam: John Benjamins.

Hatzidaki, Ourania. 1999. "'Part and Parcel': A Linguistic Analysis of Binomials and its Application to the Internal Characterization of Corpora." Unpublished Ph.D. thesis, The University of Birmingham.

Holmes, Janet. 1996. "The New Zealand spoken component of ICE: Some methodological challenges." In *Comparing English Worldwide: The International Corpus of English*, Sidney Greenbaum (ed.), 163–181. Oxford: Clarendon Press.

Holton, David, Mackridge, Peter and Philippaki-Warburton, Irene. 1997. *Greek: A Comprehensive Grammar of the Modern Language*. London: Routledge.

Horrocks, Geoffrey. 1983. "The order of constituents in Modern Greek." In *Order, Concord, and Constituency*, Gerald Gazdar, Ewan Klein and Geoffrey K. Pullum (eds), 95–111. Dordrecht: Foris Publications.

International Association for the Study of Pain. 1979. "Pain terms: A list with definitions and notes on usage." *Pain* 6: 249–252.

Inchaurralde, Carlos. 1997. "Space, reference, and emotional involvement." In *The Language of Emotions*, Susanne Niemeier and René Dirven (eds), 135–154. Amsterdam: John Benjamins.

Izard, Carroll E. 1977. *Human Emotion*. New York: Plenum Press.

Izard, Carroll E. 1992. "Basic emotions, relations among emotions, and emotion-cognition relations." *Psychological Review* 99: 561–565.

Jackendoff, Ray and Aaron, David. 1991. "Review of Lakoff and Turner (1989)." *Language* 67 (2): 320–338.

Jackson, Jean. 1992. "'After a while no one believes you': Real and unreal pain." In *Pain as Human Experience: An Anthropological Perspective*, Mary-Jo Del Veccio Good, Paul E. Brodwin, Byron J. Good and Arthur Kleinman (eds), 138–167. Berkeley: University of California Press.

Jackson, Jean. 1994. "The Rashomon approach to dealing with chronic pain." *Social Science and Medicine* 38: 823–833.

Janal, Malvin N. 1995. "Concerning the homology of painful experiences and pain descriptors: A multidimensional scaling analysis." *Pain* 64: 373–378.

Jones, Roger B. 1975/1997. "Wittgenstein's 'private language' argument." Available from: http://www.rbjones.com/rbjpub/rbjcv/papers/ugp01.htm [Accessed 20/04/2001].

Jonkers, Roel and Bastiaanse, Roelien. 1996. "The influence of instrumentality and transitivity on action naming in Broca's and anomic aphasia." *Brain and Language* 55: 37–39.

Jonkers, Roel and Bastiaanse, Roelien. 1998. "How selective are selective word class deficits? Two case studies of action and object naming." *Aphasiology* 12: 193–206.

Kenny, Anthony John Patrick. 1973. *Wittgenstein*. London: Penguin.

Kenny, Anthony John Patrick. 1994. *The Wittgenstein Reader*. Oxford: Blackwell.

Kern, Steven E. 1987. "Cultural-historical aspects of pain." *Acta Neurochirurgica* 38: 165–181.

Kidron, Yael and Kuzar, Ron. 2002. "My face is paling against my will. Emotion and control in English and Hebrew." *Pragmatics and Cognition* 10 (1–2): 129–157.

Kim, Mikyong and Thompson, Cynthia K. 2000. "Patterns of comprehension and production of nouns and verbs in agrammatism: Implications for lexical organization." *Brain and Language* 74: 1–25.

Kleinman, Arthur. 1988. *The Illness Narratives: Suffering, Healing and the Human Condition*. New York: Basic Books.

Kleinman, Arthur. 1996. "Suffering, ethics and the politics of moral life." *Culture, Medicine and Psychiatry* 20: 287–290.

Kövecses, Zoltán. 1990. *Emotion Concepts*. Berlin: Springer.

Kövecses, Zoltán. 1995. *Language and Emotion Concepts*. Duisburg: LAUD, Series A, No. 350.

Kövecses, Zoltán. 2000. *Metaphor and Emotion: Language, Culture, and Body in Human Feeling*. Cambridge: Cambridge University Press.

Kövecses, Zoltán. 2005. *Metaphor in Culture: Universality and Variation*. Cambridge: Cambridge University Press.

Kövecses, Zoltán. forth. "The conceptual structure of happiness and pain." In *Reconstructing Pain and Joy: Linguistic, Literary, and Cultural Perspectives*, Chryssoula Lascaratou, Anna Despotopoulou and Elly Ifantidou (eds), Newcastle, UK: Cambridge Scholars Publishing.

Kripke, Saul A. 1982. *Wittgenstein on Rules and Private Language: An Elementary Exposition*. Oxford: Basil Blackwell.

Kugelmann, Robert. 1999. "Complaining about chronic pain." *Social Science and Medicine* 49: 1663–1676.

Lakoff, George. 1990. "The invariance hypothesis: Is abstract reason based on image schemas?" *Cognitive Linguistics* 1 (1): 39–74.

Lakoff, George. 1993. "The contemporary theory of metaphor." In *Metaphor and Thought*, Andrew Ortony (ed.), 2nd ed. 202–251. Cambridge: Cambridge University Press.

Lakoff, George. 1996. "Sorry, I'm not myself today: The metaphor system for conceptualizing the self." In *Spaces, Worlds, and Grammar*, Gilles Fauconnier and Eve Sweetser (eds), 91–123. Chicago: The University of Chicago Press.

Lakoff, George and Johnson, Mark. 1981. "Conceptual metaphor in everyday language." In *Philosophical Perspectives on Metaphor*, Mark Johnson (ed.), 286–325. Minneapolis: University of Minnesota Press.

Lakoff, George and Johnson, Mark. 1999. *Philosophy in the Flesh: The Embodied Mind and its Challenge to Western Thought*. New York: Basic Books.

Langacker, Ronald. 1975. "Functional stratigraphy." In *Papers from the Parasession on Functionalism*, Robin E. Grossman, L. James San, and Timothy J. Vance (eds), 351–397. Chicago: Chicago Linguistic Society.

Langacker, Ronald. 1987. *Foundations of Cognitive Grammar*, Vol. 1, *Theoretical Prerequisites*. Stanford: Stanford University Press.

Langacker, Ronald. 1991. *Foundations of Cognitive Grammar*, Vol. 2, *Descriptive Applications*. Stanford: Stanford University Press.

Lascaratou, Chryssoula. 1984. "The Passive Voice in Modern Greek." Unpublished Ph.D. thesis, University of Reading.

Lascaratou, Chryssoula. 1989. *A Functional Approach to Constituent Order with Particular Reference to Modern Greek. Implications for Language Learning and Language Teaching.* Parousia Journal Monograph Series 5. Athens.

Lascaratou, Chryssoula. 1998. "Basic characteristics of Modern Greek word order." In *Constituent Order in the Languages of Europe*, Anna Siewierska (ed.), 151–171. Berlin: Mouton de Gruyter.

Lascaratou, Chryssoula and Hatzidaki, Ourania. 2002. "Pain as process in Modern Greek." *Journal of Greek Linguistics* 3: 53–82.

Lascaratou, Chryssoula and Marmaridou, Sophia. 2005. "Metaphor in Greek pain-constructions: Cognitive and functional perspectives." In *Reviewing Linguistic Thought: Converging Trends for the 21st Century*, Sophia Marmaridou, Kiki Nikiforidou and Eleni Antonopoulou (eds), 235–254. Berlin: Mouton de Gruyter.

Lascaratou, Chryssoula. forth. "The function of language in the expression of pain." In *Reconstructing Pain and Joy: Linguistic, Literary, and Cultural Perspectives*, Chryssoula Lascaratou, Anna Despotopoulou and Elly Ifantidou (eds), Newcastle, UK: Cambridge Scholars Publishing.

LeDoux, Joseph. 1998. *The Emotional Brain: The Mysterious Underpinnings of Emotional Life.* London: Phoenix.

Leder, Drew. 1990. *The Absent Body.* Chicago: University of Chicago Press.

Levin, Beth and Rappaport Hovav, Malka. 1995. *Unaccusativity: At the Syntax – Lexical Semantics Interface.* Cambridge, Mass.: The MIT Press. Linguistic Inquiry Monographs 26.

Levinas, Emmanuel. 1988. "Useless suffering." In *The Provocation of Levinas*, Robert Bernasconi and David Wood (eds), 156–167. New York: Routledge.

Levinas, Emmanuel. 1991. *Otherwise than Being or Beyond Essence.* Dordrecht: Kluwer Academic Publishers.

Marmaridou, Sophia A. S. 1984. "The Study of Reference, Attribution and Genericness in the Context of English and their Grammaticalization in M. Greek Noun Phrases." Unpublished Ph.D. thesis, University of Cambridge.

Matthiessen, Christian. 1993. "The object of study in cognitive science in relation to its construal and enactment in language." *Cultural Dynamics* 6 (1–2): 187–242.

Matthiessen, Christian. 1995a. "Theme as an enabling resource in ideational 'knowledge' construction." In *Thematic Development in English Texts*, Mohsen Ghadessy (ed.), 20–54. London: Pinter.

Matthiessen, Christian. 1995b. *Lexicogrammatical Cartography: English* Systems. Tokyo: International Language Sciences Publishers.

McBurney, Donald H. 1994. *Research Methods.* California: Brooks/Cole.

McCaffery, Margo. 1972. *Nursing Management of the Patient with Pain.* Philadelphia: Lippincott.

Melzack, Ronald. 1975. "The McGill Pain Questionnaire: Major properties and scoring methods." *Pain* 1: 277–299.

Melzack, Ronald. 1993. "Pain: Past, present and future." *Canadian Journal of Experimental Psychology* 47 (4): 615–629. Available from: http://www.alternatives.com/raven/cpain/MELZACK2.HTML [Accessed 15/09/2000].

Melzack, Ronald and Torgerson, Warren S. 1971. "On the language of pain." *Anaesthesiology* 34: 50–59.

Melzack, Ronald and Wall, Patrick D. 1988. *The Challenge of Pain*. London: Penguin.

Merskey, Harold. 1964. "An investigation of Pain in Psychological Illness." DM thesis, Oxford.

Merskey, Harold (ed.). 1986. "Classification of chronic pain: Descriptions of chronic pain syndromes and definitions of pain terms." *Pain* 24, Suppl. 1.

Merskey, Harold. 1994. "Logic, truth and language in concepts of pain." *Quality of Life Research* 3 (1): S69–S76.

Morris, David B. 1991. *The Culture of Pain*. Berkeley: University of California Press.

Moser, Amalia. 1993. "Γραμματικοποίηση και βοηθητικά ρήματα." *Studies in Greek Linguistics* 14: 161–175.

Nakas, Thanassis and Gavriilidou, Zoe. 2005. *Δημοσιογραφία και Νεολογία* [Journalism and Neologism]. Athens: Patakis Publishers.

Niemeier, Susanne. 1997. "Introduction." In *The Language of Emotions*, Susanne Niemeier and René Dirven (eds), vii-xviii. Amsterdam: John Benjamins.

Niemeier, Susanne and Dirven, René (eds). 1997. *The Language of Emotions*. Amsterdam: John Benjamins.

Nikiforidou, Kiki. 1991. "The meaning of the genitive: A case study in semantic structure and semantic change." *Cognitive Linguistics* 2 (2): 149–205.

Nikiforidou, Kiki. 1999. "Η μεταφορικότητα της σκέψης: Φιλοσοφικές και γλωσσολογικές προσεγγίσεις." In *Γλώσσα και Νόηση* [Language and Cognition], Dimitra Kati, Marianna Kondyli and Kiki Nikiforidou (eds), 163–178. Athens: Ekdoseis Alexandria.

Nissenbaum, Helen Fay. 1985. *Emotion and Focus*. Stanford: CSLI.

Norvell, Kristine Turner, Gaston-Johansson, Fannie and Zimmerman, Lani. 1990. "Pain description by nurses and physicians." *Journal of Pain and Symptom Management* 5 (1): 11–17.

Omondi, Lucia N. 1997. "Dholuo emotional language: An overview." In *The Language of Emotions*, Susanne Niemeier and René Dirven (eds), 87–109. Amsterdam: John Benjamins.

Papageorgiou, Ann C. and Badley, Elizabeth M. 1989. "The quality of pain in arthritis: The words patients use to describe overall pain and pain in individual joints at rest and on movement." *Journal of Rheumatology* 16 (1): 106–112.

Paulson, Margareta, Danielson, Ella and Söderberg, Siv. 2002. "Struggling for a tolerable existence: The meaning of men's lived experiences of living with pain of fibromyalgia type." *Qualitative Health Research* 12 (2): 238–249.

Pavlenko, Aneta. 2002. "Emotions and the body in Russian and English." *Pragmatics and Cognition* 10 (1–2): 207–241.

Peters, Hans. 2004. "The vocabulary of pain." In *Categorization in the History of English*, Christian J. Kay and Jeremy J. Smith (eds), 193–220. Amsterdam: John Benjamins.

Philippaki-Warburton, Irene. 1985. "Word order in Modern Greek." *Transactions of the Philological Society*: 113–143.

Philippaki-Warburton, Irene. 1987. "The theory of empty categories and the pro-drop parameter in Modern Greek." *Journal of Linguistics* 23: 289–318.

Philippaki-Warburton, Irene. 1992. *Εισαγωγή στη Θεωρητική Γλωσσολογία* [Introduction to Theoretical Linguistics]. Athens: Nefeli.

Pincus, Tamar, Pearce, Shirley and Perrott, Alisa. 1996. "Pain patients' bias in the interpretation of ambiguous homophones." *British Journal of Medical Psychology* 69: 259–266.

Poole, Garry D. and Craig, Kenneth D. 1992. "Judgements of genuine, suppressed and faked facial expressions of pain." *Journal of Personal and Social Psychology* 63: 797–805.

Rey, Roselyn. 1993/1998. *The History of Pain*. Massachusetts: Harvard University Press.

Rosaldo, Michelle Z. 1984. "Toward an anthropology of self and feeling." In *Culture Theory: Essays on Mind, Self, and Emotion*, Richard A. Shweder and Robert A. LeVine (eds), 137–157. Cambridge: Cambridge University Press.

Scarry, Elaine. 1985. *The Body in Pain: The Making and Unmaking of the World*. New York: Oxford University Press.

Schweizer, Harold. 1995. "To give suffering a language." *Literature and Medicine* 14 (2): 210–221.

Semino, Elena, Heywood, John and Short, Mick. 2004. "Methodological problems in the analysis of metaphors in a corpus of conversations about cancer." *Journal of Pragmatics* 36: 1271–1294.

Sinclair, John McHardy. 1991. *Corpus, Concordance, Collocation*. Oxford: Oxford University Press.

Sinclair, John McHardy. 1994. "Corpus Typology: A Framework for Classification." Birmingham: Eagles Report 080294.

Smith, M. C. 1992. "Metaphor in nursing theory." *Nursing Science Quarterly* 5: 48–49.

Solomon, Robert C. 1995. "The crosscultural comparison of emotion." In *Emotions in Asian Thought*, Joel Marks and Roger T. Ames (eds), 253–308. Albany: State University of New York Press.

Söderberg, Siv and Norberg, Astrid. 1995. "Metaphorical pain language among fibromyalgia patients." *Scandinavian Journal of Caring Sciences* 9: 55–59.

Sontag, Susan. 1991. *Illness as Metaphor: AIDS and its Metaphors*. London: Penguin.

Talmy, Len. 1988. "Force dynamics in language and cognition." *Cognitive Science* 12: 49–100.

The Compact Oxford English Dictionary. 1991. 2nd ed. Oxford: Clarendon Press.

Theodoropoulou, Maria. 1999. "Γλώσσα και συναίσθημα: Τα αντικείμενα του φόβου." In *Γλώσσα και Νόηση* [Language and Cognition], Dimitra Kati, Marianna Kondyli and Kiki Nikiforidou (eds), 207–223. Athens: Ekdoseis Alexandria.

Theodoropoulou, Maria. 2004. *Στα Γλωσσικά Μονοπάτια του Φόβου: Ψυχισμός και Γλώσσα* [Treading the Linguistic Paths of Fear: Psyche and Language]. Athens: Nisos.

Theodoropoulou, Maria. forth. "Metaphors of joy and happiness in Greek: The case of positive emotions." In *Reconstructing Pain and Joy: Linguistic, Literary, and Cultural Perspectives*, Chryssoula Lascaratou, Anna Despotopoulou and Elly Ifantidou (eds), Newcastle, UK: Cambridge Scholars Publishing.

Theophanopoulou-Kontou, Dimitra. 1988. "Δομές της σύνθετης ΟΦ και μετακίνηση στην ΝΕ." *Studies in Greek Linguistics* 9: 337–354.

Theophanopoulou-Kontou, Dimitra. 1999. "Δομές με προοπτική του δέκτη και η κατανομή του -ω/-μαι: Τα αντιμεταβιβαστικά και παθητικά." *Studies in Greek Linguistics* 20: 146–157.

Thomas, Jenny and Wilson, Andrew. 1996. "Methodologies for studying a corpus of doctor-patient interaction." In *Using Corpora for Language Research*, Jenny Thomas and Mick Short (eds), 92–109. London: Longman.

Thompson, Cynthia K., Lange, K. L., Schneider, Sandra L. and Shapiro, Lewis P. 1997. "Agrammatic and non-brain-damaged subjects' verb and verb argument structure production." *Aphasiology* 11: 473–490.

Toombs, Kay S. 1993. *The Meaning of Illness*. Dordrecht: Kluwer.

Tsimpli, Ianthi-Maria. 1990. "The clause structure and word order of Modern Greek." *UCL Working Papers in Linguistics* 2: 226–255.

Tzartzanos, Achileas. 1946/1963. *Νεοελληνική Σύνταξις* [Modern Greek Syntax], 2nd ed. Vol. 1. Athens: Organismos Ekdoseos Scholikon Vivlion.

Tzavaras, Thanasis. 1999. "Σημειώσεις περί μητρικής γλώσσας από ψυχαναλυτική κυρίως άποψη." In *Γλώσσα και Νόηση* [Language and Cognition], Dimitra Kati, Marianna Kondyli and Kiki Nikiforidou (eds), 239–246. Athens: Ekdoseis Alexandria.

Veloudis, Ioannis. 2003. "Possession and conversation: The case of the category perfect." In *Perfect Explorations*, Artemis Alexiadou, Monika Rathert and Arnim von Stechow (eds), 381–399. Berlin: Mouton de Gruyter.

Waddie, Nicola A. 1996. "Language and pain expression." *Journal of Advanced Nursing* 23: 868–872.

Wall, Patrick D. and Melzack, Ronald (eds). 1989. *Textbook of Pain*, 2nd ed. Edinburgh: Churchill Livingstone.

Walters, A. 1963. "The psychological aspects of bodily pain." *Applied Therapy* 5: 853–856.

Watson, Jean. 1987. "Nursing on the caring edge: Metaphorical vignettes." *Advanced Nursing Science* 10: 10–18.

Wierzbicka, Anna. 1980. *Lingua Mentalis: The Semantics of Natural Language*. Sydney: Academic Press.

Wierzbicka, Anna. 1988. *The Semantics of Grammar*. Amsterdam: John Benjamins.

Wierzbicka, Anna. 1992. *Semantics, Culture and Cognition: Universal Human Concepts in Culture-Specific Configurations*. New York: Oxford University Press.

Wierzbicka, Anna. 1995a. "Everyday conceptions of emotions: A semantic perspective." In *Everyday Conceptions of Emotions: An Introduction to the Psychology, Anthropology and Linguistics of Emotions*, James Russell et al. (eds), 17–47. Dordrecht: Kluwer.

Wierzbicka, Anna. 1995b. "The relevance of language to the study of emotions." Paper read at the 21st LAUD Symposium on 'The Language of Emotions' (Duisburg, 10–11 April 1995).

Wierzbicka, Anna. 1996. *Semantics: Primes and Universals*. Oxford: Oxford University Press.

Wierzbicka, Anna. 1997. *Understanding Cultures through their Key Words. English, Russian, Polish, German, and Japanese*. New York: Oxford University Press.

Wierzbicka, Anna. 1999. *Emotions across Languages and Cultures: Diversity and Universals*. Cambridge: Cambridge University Press.

Wittgenstein, Ludwig. 1953/1989. *Philosophical Investigations*. Oxford: Basil Blackwell.

Wittgenstein, Ludwig. 1969/1974. *Philosophical Grammar*. Oxford: Basil Blackwell.

Appendix A: Pain as process

Mapping Greek 'pain' expressions onto Halliday's paradigm of English ones

		(a) 'pain' expression	freq.	%	(bi) type of process	(bii) structural functions	(c) agnate expression
1	Gr	**to xeri mu ponai** the arm-NOM my hurt-PRS:3SG 'my arm hurts'	39	4.36	relational: attributive	body part = Carrier; Attribute / Process	**i mustarδa kei** the mustard-NOM burn-PRS:3SG **(ine kafteri)** (is-PRS:3SG hot-NOM) 'the mustard is hot'
	En	my arm hurts / aches					the paint sticks ('is sticky')
2	Gr	**to xeri mu ponai** the arm-NOM my hurt-PRS:3SG 'my arm's hurting'	30	3.35	material: middle [existential: occurring]	body part = Medium [body part = Setting]	**ta xeria mu tremun** the hand-PL:NOM my shake-PRS:3PL 'my hands are shaking' **[to tavani stazi]** the roof-NOM leak-PRS:3SG 'the roof's leaking'
	En	my arm's hurting / aching					my nose is bleeding [the roof's leaking]
(1+2) a		**(to xeri mu) ponai**	53	5.92			

		(a) 'pain' expression	freq.	%	(bi) type of process	(bii) structural functions	(c) agnate expression
(1+2) b		**(to xeri mu) mu ponai** (the arm-NOM my) I-GEN hurt-PRS:3SG '(my arm) it hurts / is hurting (in) me'	10	1.11			**(ta poδja mu) mu muδjazun** (the feet-NOM my) I-GEN numb-PRS:3PL '(my feet) they get / are getting numb'
3	Gr	**ponao (eδo)** hurt-PRS:1SG (here) 'I hurt (here)'	101	11.28	relational: attributive [behavioural]	person = Carrier; Attribute / Process [person = Behaver]	**simpasxo** sympathise-PRS:1SG 'I sympathise' **[anisixo]** worry-PRS:1SG 'I worry'
	En	I hurt / ache (here)					I sympathise [I grieve, I worry]
3a		**ponas (eδo)?** hurt-PRS:2SG (here) 'do you hurt (here)?'	111	12.40			

		(a) 'pain' expression	freq.	%	(bi) type of process	(bii) structural functions	(c) agnate expression
4	Gr	**ponao (eδo)** hurt-PRS:1SG (here) 'I'm hurting (here)'	106	11.84	material: middle [existential: occurring] [behavioural]	person = Medium [person = Setting] [person = Behaver]	**emoraγo** bleed-PRS:1SG 'I'm bleeding' [**kriono**] feel-cold-PRS:1SG 'I'm feeling cold' [**tremo**] tremble / shake-PRS:1SG 'I'm trembling / shaking'
	En	I'm hurting / aching (here)					I'm bleeding [I'm peeling, I'm trembling]
4a		**ponas (eδo)?** hurt-PRS:2SG (here) 'are you hurting (here)?'	101	11.28			
5	Gr	**ponai (eδo)** hurt-PRS:3SG:IMPERS (here) 'it hurts (here)'	21	2.35	existential: existing	impersonal Setting	**γlistrai (eδo)** slip-PRS:3SG:impers (here) 'it is slippery (here)'
	En	it hurts / aches (here)					it echoes

		(a) 'pain' expression	freq.	%	(bi) type of process	(bii) structural functions	(c) agnate expression
6	Gr	**ponai (eδo)** hurt-PRS:3SG:IMPERS (here) 'it's hurting (here)'	155	17.32	existential: occurring	impersonal Setting	**vrexi** rain-PRS:3SG:IMPERS 'it's raining' **xionizi** snow-PRS:3SG:IMPERS 'it's snowing'
	En	it's hurting / aching (here)					it's raining
7	Gr	**to xeri mu me ponai** the arm-NOM my I-ACC hurt-PRS:3SG 'my arm's hurting me'	27	3.02	mental: impacting	body part = Phenomenon / Agent; person = Senser	**i zesti me pirazi** the heat-NOM I-ACC bother-PRS:3SG 'the heat's bothering me'
	En	my arm's hurting me					the heat's bothering me
7a		**(to xeri mu) me ponai**	27	3.02			
8	Gr	**me ponas** I-ACC hurt-PRS:2SG 'you're hurting me'	8	0.89	material: effective	person = Goal; other (person / object) = Actor	**me patas** I-ACC tread-PRS:2SG 'you're treading on me (my toes)'
	En	you're hurting me					you're pushing me

		(a) 'pain' expression	freq.	%	(bi) type of process	(bii) structural functions	(c) agnate expression
9	Gr	**xtipisa to xeri mu** hit-PST:1SG the arm-ACC my 'I've hurt my arm' *[not extracted from the data]*	0	0.0	material: effective	person = Actor; body part = Goal	**eskisa to pandeloni mu** tear-PST:1SG the pants-ACC my 'I've torn my pants'
	En	I've hurt my arm					I've broken my glasses
10	Gr	**xtipisa (sto xeri mu)** hit-PST:1SG (in-the arm-ACC my) 'I've hurt myself (on the arm)' *[not extracted from the data]*	0	0.0	material: effective / reflexive	person = Actor; body part = Location	**kopika** cut-PST:PASS:1SG 'I've cut myself' **kaika** burn-PST:PASS:1SG 'I've burnt myself'
	En	I've hurt myself (on the arm)					I've ruined myself

		(a) 'pain' expression	freq.	%	(bi) type of process	(bii) structural functions	(c) agnate expression
11	Gr	**afto ponai** that-NOM hurt-PRS:3SG 'that hurts'	26	2.90	mental [relational: attributive / agentive]	(object / process) = Phenomenon [Attribute/ Process; other (object / process) = Agent]	**afto enoxli** that-NOM annoy-PRS:3SG 'that annoys' [**afto leroni**] that-NOM dirty-PRS:3SG 'that dirties'
	En	that hurts					that dirties ('causes things to be dirty')
12	Gr	**afto me ponai** that-NOM I-ACC hurt-PRS:3SG 'that's hurting me'	16	1.79	material: effective	person = Goal; other (object / process) = Actor	**afto me tsimbai** that-NOM I-ACC prick-PRS:3SG 'that's pricking me' **afto me γarγalai** that-NOM I-ACC tickle-PRS:3SG 'that's tickling me'
12a	Gr	**(afto) me ponai**	5	0.56			

		(a) 'pain' expression	freq.	%	(bi) type of process	(bii) structural functions	(c) agnate expression
13	Gr	**me ponai (eδo)** I-ACC hurt-PRS:3SG: IMPERS (here) 'it hurts me (here)'	21	2.35	mental: effective	person = Senser other = impersonal Phenomenon	**me tsuzi (eδo)** I-ACC sting-PRS:3SG IMPERS (here) 'it stings me (here)'
14	Gr	**me ponai (eδo)** I-ACC hurt-PRS:3SG: IMPERS (here) 'it's hurting me (here)'	38	4.24	mental: impacting		**me troi (eδo)** I-ACC itch-PRS:3SG:IMPERS (here) 'it's itching me (here)'
		TOTAL	895	100.0			

Appendix B: Pain as thing

Mapping Greek 'pain' expressions onto Halliday's paradigm of English ones

		(a) 'pain' expression	(bi) type of process	(bii) structural functions	(c) agnate expression
15	Gr	**exo (enan) pono sti mesi** have-PRS:1SG pain-ACC in-the low-back-ACC 'I've got (a) pain in the / my low back'	relational: attributive / possessive	'pain' = Attribute (possessed); person = Carrier	**exo (ena) sinaxi** have-PRS:1SG cold-in-the-head-ACC 'I've got a cold in the head'
	En	I've got a headache / a pain in my neck			I've got a chest cold
16	Gr	**afto mu δini / ferni / prokali / kani ponokefalo** this-NOM I-GEN give / bring / cause / make-PRS:3SG headache 'that gives me a headache'	relational: attributive / possessive / agentive	(as no. 15); other (object / process) = Agent	**afto mu ferni ipno / nista** this-NOM I-GEN bring-PRS:3SG sleep / sleepiness-ACC 'that makes me sleepy' **afto mu δini xara / efxaristisi** this-NOM I-GEN give-PRS:3SG joy / pleasure-ACC 'that gives me joy / pleasure' **afto mu prokali meγali θlipsi / ekpliksi** this-NOM I-GEN cause-PRS:3SG great sorrow / surprise-ACC 'that causes great sorrow / surprise to me'
	En	that gives me a headache			that gives me a thought

		(a) 'pain' expression	(bi) type of process	(bii) structural functions	(c) agnate expression
17	Gr	**afto mu δini / ferni / prokali / kani ponokefalo** this-NOM I-GEN give / bring / cause / make-PRS:3SG headache 'that's giving me a headache'	material: effective: benefactive	'pain' = Goal; person = Beneficiary; other = Actor	**afto mu ferni ipno / nista** this-NOM I-GEN bring-PRS:3SG sleep / sleepiness-ACC 'that's making me sleepy' **afto mu δini xara / efxaristisi** this-NOM I-GEN give-PRS:3SG joy / pleasure-ACC 'that's giving me joy / pleasure' **afto mu prokali meγali θlipsi / ekpliksi** this-NOM I-GEN cause-PRS:3SG great sorrow / surprise-ACC 'that's causing great sorrow / surprise to me'
	En	that's giving me a headache			that's giving me a lot of help
18	Gr	**njoθis eki pono?** feel-PRS:2SG there pain-ACC 'do you feel (any) pain there?'	mental: scope-defining	'pain' = Phenomenon; person = Senser	**akus θorivo?** hear-PRS:2SG noise-ACC 'do you hear (any) noise?' **vlepis fos?** see-PRS:2SG light-ACC 'do you see (any) light?'
	En	do you feel any pain?			do you see any smoke?

		(a) 'pain' expression	(bi) type of process	(bii) structural functions	(c) agnate expression
19	Gr	**o ponos mu ine avastaxtos ti nixta** the pain-NOM my be-PRS:3SG intolerable the night-ACC 'my pain is intolerable at night'	relational: attributive	'pain' = Carrier; quality = Attribute	**i elpiδes mu ine lijes / i aγonia mu ine meγali** the hopes-NOM my be-PRS:3PL few-NOM / the suspense-NOM my be-PRS:3SG great-NOM 'my hopes are few' / 'my suspense is great'
	En	my pain is bad today			my hopes are high
20	En	are you in (great) pain?	relational: attributive / circumstantial	'pain' = (circumstantial) Attribute; person = Carrier	are you in great suspense?
	Gr	[*no directly corresponding Greek ponos construction, despite the possibility of agnate expressions of emotions*]			**ise se (meγali) aγonia / anisixia?** be-PRS:2SG in great suspense / distress-ACC 'are you in (great) suspense / distress?'

		(a) 'pain' expression	(bi) type of process	(bii) structural functions	(c) agnate expression
21	Gr	**o ponos ipoδiloni / δixni oti…** the pain-NOM suggest / show-PRS:3SG (that) 'the pain suggests / shows that…' [*not extracted from the data*]	verbal	'pain' = Sayer	**i iγrasia δixni oti…** the damp-NOM show-PRS:3SG that 'the damp suggests that…' **o piretos δixni oti…** the fever-NOM show-PRS:3SG that 'the fever suggests / indicates that…'
	En	the pain suggests (that)…			the damp suggests that…
22	Gr	**to 10 ine o aforitos ponos** the 10 be-PRS:3SG the excruciating pain-NOM 'score 10 is / represents the excruciating pain'	relational: identifying	score = Identifier/ Token 'pain' = Identified/ Value	**o vaθmos 20 ine to "arista"** the grade-NOM 20 be-PRS:3SG the excellent-NOM 'grade 20 is "excellent"'
23	Gr	**ine enas ponos eδo** be-PRS:3SG a pain-NOM here 'there is (a) pain here'	existential: existing	'pain' = Existent	**ine enas aγnostos sto γrafio** be-PRS:3SG a stranger-NOM in-the office-ACC 'there is a stranger in the office'

Appendix C

Typical corpus dialogues presented in full

1. Private physiotherapy clinic. Dialogue No 6

P: …i γrami… afti i γrami.
the line-NOM this the line-NOM
'…the line… this line.'

D: i γrami… se ponai eki?
the line-NOM you-ACC hurt-PRS:3SG:IMPERS there
'The line… Does it hurt you there?'

P: mm.
mm
'Mm.'

D: mm?
mm
'Mm?'

P: oxi. apo eδo δen ponai. apo eδo pera, kseris, anakufizome. ama θelo n' anakufisto jirizo apo eδo.
no from here not hurt-PRS:3SG:IMPERS from here over know-PRS:2SG get-relief-PRS:1SG when want-PRS:1SG to-PARTCL get-relief-PFV:NON-PST:1SG turn-PRS:1SG from here
'No. It doesn't hurt on this side. On this side, you know, I get some relief. When I want to get some relief I turn on this side.'

D: ne, ne. kamburjase liγo. kamburjase. mi, min alazis θesi… xalarose, re x.
yes yes bend-IMP:2SG a-little bend-IMP:2SG not not change-IMP:2SG position-ACC relax-IMP:2SG you
'Yes, yes. Bend a little. Bend. Don't, don't change position… relax, you.'

P: apo eki arxizi ke ponai.
from there start-PRS:3SG:IMPERS and hurt-PRS:3SG:IMPERS
'It starts hurting from that position.'

D: (She laughs.)

P: ax, kale, ponai!!! (He is a man, but he speaks like a woman here.)
ah dear hurt-PRS:3SG:IMPERS
'Oh, dear, it's hurting!!!'

D: (She laughs.) ela, vre x. stasu… ela liɣo pjo piso.
come-on-IMP:2SG man hold-on-IMP:2SG come-IMP:2SG a-bit further back
'Come on, you. Hold on… Move a bit further back.'

P: proti fora xtes to vraδi δe borusa na kratiso to kefali mu. eprepe na to kratao. δe borusa na to stirikso.
first time-ACC yesterday the evening-ACC not can-PST:1SG to-PARTCL hold-PFV:NON-PST:1SG the head-ACC my must-PST to-PARTCL it-ACC hold-PRS:1SG not can-PST:1SG to-PARTCL it-ACC support-PFV:NON-PST:1SG
'For the first time last evening I couldn't keep my head upright. I had to hold it myself. I couldn't keep it upright.'

D: ja pame pali. jirna… eki pai, etsi?
just go-IMP:1PL again turn-around-IMP:2SG there go-PRS:3SG like-this
'Let's go again. Turn around… it moves as far as that, doesn't it?'

P: ne.
yes
'Yes.'

D: ine ke o mis, ala prepi na ine ke i arθrosi. ja jirna… i arθrosi.
be-PRS:3SG and the muscle-NOM but must-PRS to-PARTCL be-PRS:3SG and the joint-NOM just turn-around-IMP:2SG the joint-NOM
'It's also the muscle, but it must be the joint too. Just turn around… the joint.'

P: a! ponai. aman! 29 ores! ores anamonis sto amsterdam… pjo poli eδo.
ouch hurt-PRS:3SG:IMPERS my-goodness 29 hours hours of-waiting in-the Amsterdam more here
'Ouch! It's hurting. My goodness! 29 hours! Hours waiting in Amsterdam… more here.'

D: ne, ne, pjo poli… stasu na δo. xalarose.
yes yes more stay-IMP:2SG to-PARTCL see-PFV:NON-PST:1SG relax-IMP:2SG
'Yes, yes, even more… let me see. Relax.'

P: mmm! o! aau, aau, aau! au!
mmm ouch ouch ouch ouch ouch
'Mmm! Ouch! Ouch, ouch, ouch, ouch!'

D: eδo njoθis na… kaθolu?
here feel-PRS:2SG to-PARTCL at-all
'Here do you feel that it… at all?'

P: eki, oxi, oxi, oxi. kato, kato ap' tin omoplati, apo kato.
there no no no under under from the shoulder-blade-ACC from under
'There, no, no, no. Below, below the shoulder blade, below.'

D: …tin omoplati. apo kato ap' tin omoplati.
the shoulder-blade-ACC from under from the shoulder-blade-ACC
'…the shoulder blade. Below the shoulder blade.'

P: …eki! au! eki, eki!
there ouch there there
'…there! Ouch! There, there!

D: …oxi, eδo ine i omoplati.
no here be-PRS:3SG the shoulder-blade-NOM
'…no, it's the shoulder blade here.'

P: e, endaksi, apo kato su leo, o mis…
eh all-right from under you-GEN tell-PRS:1SG the muscle-NOM
'Well, all right, I mean below, the muscle…'

D: eδo.
here
'Here.'

P: eδo.
here
'Here.'

D: kitakse, i omoplati ine…
look-IMP:2SG the shoulder-blade-NOM be-PRS:3SG
'Look, it's the shoulder blade…'

P: katse na su δikso…
sit-IMP:2SG to-PARTCL you-GEN show-PFV:NON-PST:1SG
'Let me show you…'

D: ksero pu ine!
know-PRS:1SG where be-PRS:3SG
'I know where it is!'

P: oxi, otan leo apo kato ine… pos… sa na vazis to xeri apo kato, eδo. prepi na exi ena sinδezmo eki…
no when say-PRS:1SG from under be-PRS:3SG how like to PARTCL put-PRS:2SG the hand-ACC from under here must-PRS to-PARTCL exist-PRS:3SG:IMPERS one ligament-ACC there
'No, when I say it's below… how… as if you are putting your hand below, here. There must be a ligament there…'

D: δen ine…
not be-PRS:3SG
'It is not…'

P: bravo!
well-done
'That's it!'

D: ...ine enas mis eki...
be-PRS:3SG:IMPERS a muscle-NOM there
'...there's a muscle there...'

P: eδo, eδo ponai, eδo ponao.
here here hurt-PRS:3SG:IMPERS here hurt-PRS:1SG
'Here, it's hurting here, I'm hurting here.'

D: kitakse, ponai ki eδo. apo kato.
look-IMP:2SG hurt-PRS:3SG:IMPERS and here from under
'Look, it's hurting here, too. Below.'

P: ne, apo kato. afto su leo, apo kato. fere ton papu eδo na su δixni.
yes from under this-ACC you-GEN tell-PRS:1SG from under bring-IMP:2SG the grandfather-ACC here to-PARTCL you-GEN show-PRS:3SG
'Yes, below. That's what I'm telling you, below. Get grandfather here to show you.'

D: aftos o atimos o...
this the nasty-NOM the-NOM
'That nasty...'

P: au! eki! vlepis, eki pu exis ton andixira.
ouch there see-PRS:2SG there where have-PRS:2SG the thumb-NOM
'Ouch! There! See, where your thumb is.'

D: mmm...
mmm
'Mmm...'

P: au!
ouch
'Ouch!'

D: o ano trapezoiδis, e, o opisθios oδondotos.
the upper trapezius-NOM eh the serratus anterior-NOM
'The upper trapezius (muscle), eh, the serratus anterior (muscle).'

P: eki, eki.
there there
'There, there.'

D: to kefali su...
the head-NOM your
'Your head...'

P: ...pu γrafis anastenaγmata ke θa nomisi ala praγmata...
that record-PRS:2SG sighs-ACC and will think-PFV:NON-PST:2SG other things-ACC
'...you are recording sighs and she will imagine other things...'

D: (She laughs.) les?! ba! ja stripse tora.
say-PRS:2SG no-way just turn-IMP:2SG now
'Do you think so? No way! Just turn now.'

P: ponao!… eδo ponai. liγotero. ama to voiθas etsi δen ponai toso poli. ponai.
hurt-PRS:1SG here hurt-PRS:3SG:IMPERS less when it-ACC help-PRS:2SG like-this not hurt-PRS:3SG:IMPERS so much hurt-PRS:3SG:IMPERS
'I'm hurting!… It's hurting here. Less. When you help it like this, it doesn't hurt so much. It's hurting.'

D: ponai, e?
hurt-PRS:3SG:IMPERS eh
'It's hurting, is it?'

P: eki, ne, ama pao pjo piso, ponai pjo…
there yes when go-PRS:1SG further back hurt-PRS:3SG:IMPERS more
'There, yes, when I move further back, it hurts more…'

D: stasu, stasu, s'afti ti θesi, min pas perisotero. pes mu an se ponai afto.
hold-on-IMP:2SG hold-on-IMP:2SG in this-ACC the position-ACC not go-IMP:2SG further tell-IMP:2SG I-GEN if you-ACC hurt-PRS:3SG this-NOM
'Hold on, hold on, in this position, don't move any further. Tell me if this hurts you.'

P: oxi.
no
'No.'

D: afto?
this-NOM
'This?'

P: afto ama to ekanes θa ponaje.
this-NOM if it-ACC do-IPFV:2SG will hurt-IPFV:3SG:IMPERS
'If you did this it would hurt.'

D: eδo?
here
'Here?'

P: …na strivo δen ponai.
to-PARTCL turn-PRS:1SG not hurt-PRS:3SG:IMPERS
'…when I turn it doesn't hurt.'

D: eki?
there
'There?'

P: ne, ponai apo eδo tora. au!
yes hurt-PRS:3SG:IMPERS from here now ouch
'Yes, it's hurting here now. Ouch!'

D: eki?… i mies mono. ja stripes… malon.
there the muscles-NOM only just turn-IMP:2SG probably
'There?… the muscles only. Just turn… Probably.'

P: pjo siniθis… eδo.
more usual-NOM here
'More usual… here.'

D: aku kaθaroδefterjatika na me vazi na δulevo!
listen-IMP:2SG Clean-Monday to-PARTCL I-ACC put-PRS:3SG to-PARTCL work-PRS:1SG
'Who would believe such a thing! He makes me work on Clean Monday!'

P: e, ne!
eh yes
'Eh, yes!'

D: to paljopeδo!
the old-boy-NOM
'The naughty boy!'

P: iδes! ti fteo eγo re peδaki mu an iparxun apokries ke xoreveis tis apokries…?
see-PST:2SG what be-to-blame-PRS:1SG I-NOM child-DIMIN:VOC if exist-PRS:3PL carnival-PL:NOM and dance-PRS:2SG the carnival-PL:ACC
'See! Why blame me, my friend, if there's carnival and you dance during the carnival period…?'

P: o… o… ox! eki ponai. au! mmmmjau!
oh oh oh there hurt-PRS:3SG:IMPERS ouch meow
'Oh… oh… oh! It's hurting there. Ouch! Meow!'

D: (She laughs.) ti ponos ine?
what pain-NOM be-PRS:3SG
'What (kind of) pain is it?'

P: au! θa katalavis pja ine astia ke pja sovara.
ouch will understand-PFV:NON-PST:2SG which-PL:NOM be-PRS:3PL funny-PL:NOM and which serious-PL:NOM
'Ouch! You will understand which ones are funny and which ones are serious.'

D: e, kala.
eh all-right
'Eh, all right.'

P: au, au, au, au! eki, eki, aftos δen ine kaθolu astios.
ouch ouch ouch ouch there there this-NOM not be-PRS:3SG at-all funny-NOM
'Ouch, ouch, ouch, ouch! There, there, this one is not at all funny.'

D: pos ine aftos o ponos su?
how be-PRS:3SG this the pain-NOM your
'What is this pain of yours like?'

P: ʃarp! kseris, oksitatos, eki, in'... au! au! au! eki. aaaa...!
sharp-NOM know-PRS:2SG most-sharp-NOM there be-PRS:3SG ouch ouch ouch there ouch
'"Sharp"! You know, very sharp, there, it's... Ouch! Ouch! Ouch! There. Ouch...!'

D: afto to simio akrivos ine to pjo... pjo δinatos?
this the spot-NOM exactly be-PRS:3SG the most most strong-NOM
'Is the most... the strongest one in this specific spot?'

P: au! eki, eki, eki, eki ine to pjo δinato! au! au... o... oox! kseris mja fora o oδondiatros efaγe γroθja sto stomaxi, e!
ouch there there there there be-PRS:3SG the strongest-NOM ouch ouch ouch ouch know-PRS:2SG one time-ACC the dentist-NOM get-PST:3SG punch-NOM in-the stomach-ACC eh
'Ouch! There, there, there, there is the strongest one! Ouch! Ouch... ouch... ouch! You know, the dentist got a punch in the stomach once, eh!'

D: mmm...
mmm
'Mmm...'

P: prosexe...
watch-IMP:2SG
'Watch out...'

D: e, sta poδia θa fao, δen ine tipote.
eh in-the legs-ACC will get-PFV:NON-PST:1SG not be-PRS:3SG:IMPERS nothing-NOM
'Well, I'll be punched in the legs, it's nothing.'

P: ...me perimene me tin enesi sto xeri.
I-ACC wait-IPFV:3SG with the injection-ACC in-the hand-ACC
'...he was waiting for me with the injection in his hand.'

D: (She laughs.) eγo δen exo enesi.
I-NOM not have-PRS:1SG injection-ACC
'But, I haven't got any injection.'

P: au! aaa!
ouch ouch
'Ouch! Ouch!'

D: exi malakosi liγo.
have-PRS:3SG soften-PFV a-bit
'It's a bit milder.'

P: e, ja na min urljazo, an kanis sto iδjo simio…
eh for to-PARTCL not scream-PRS:1SG if do-PRS:2SG in-the same spot-ACC
'Eh, since I'm not screaming, if you are doing it in the same spot…'

D: sto iδjo, δen alaksa.
in-the same-ACC not change-PST:1SG
'In the same one, I haven't changed.'

P: aaa! eki, eki, eki, ekiii, ekiii (singing)…
ouch there there there there there
'Ouch! There, there, there, theeere, theeere…'

D: exo kolisi to δaxtilo mu…
have-PRS:1SG stick-PFV the finger-ACC my
'I've stuck my finger…'

P: eki, eki. ke liγo pjo pano.
there there and a-bit more up
'There, there. And a bit higher up.'

D: θa pao ke pjo pano. liγo akoma eδo. eδo mu ipes pjo, oti ine pjo oksis…
will go-PRS:1SG and more up a-bit more here here I-GEN tell-PST:2SG more that be-PRS:3SG more sharp-NOM
'I'll move it even higher up. A bit more, here. You told me (that) here (it's) more, that it's sharper…'

P: nee, nee…
yes yes
'Yeah, yeah…'

D: …o ponos…
the pain-NOM
'…the pain…'

P: au! aaah! ax!
ouch ouch ouch
'Ouch! Ouch! Ouch!

D: pu se ponai tora?
where you-ACC hurt-PRS:3SG:IMPERS now
'Where is it hurting you now?'

P: e, liγotero!
eh less
'Eh, less!'

D: ftani, δen exi alo!
be-enough-PRS:3SG:IMPERS not have-PRS:3SG:IMPERS anymore
'That's enough, that's all!'

2. Metaxa Cancer Hospital, pain management clinic. Dialogue No 17

D: poso xronon iste?
how-many years-GEN be-PRS:2PL
'How old are you?'

P: 43.
43
'43.'

D: 43. ke xirurjiθikate ja to stomaxi ke ton isofaγo. ti kanate?
43 and operate-PASS:PST:2PL for the stomach-ACC and the esophagus-ACC what do-PST:2PL
'43. And you have been operated for the stomach and the esophagus. What have you done?'

P: ne.
yes
'Yes.'

D: pote?
when
'When?'

P: 21 avγustu tu 2000.
21 august-GEN the-GEN 2000
'(On) 21 August 2000.'

D: ke apo tote? ponate apo tote?
and since then hurt-PRS:2PL since then
'And since then? Have you been hurting since then?'

P: ...ponao... sinexja.
hurt-PRS:1SG continuously
'...I have been hurting... continuously.'

D: pu ta kanate ola afta?
where do-PST:2PL all these-NOM
'Where have you done all this?'

P: ston evangelizmo.
at-the Evangelismos-ACC
'At Evangelismos (Hospital).'

D: mmm... borite ke trote?
mmm can-PRS:2PL and eat-PRS:2PL
'Mmm... Can you eat?'

P: oxi.
no
'No.'

D: pu ponate akrivos?
where hurt-PRS:2PL exactly
'Where exactly do you hurt?'

P: ...afto...
this-NOM
'...this...'

D: i kilia... ne.
the belly-NOM yes
'The belly... Yes.'

P: eδo me ponese poli...
here I-ACC hurt-PST:3SG:IMPERS a-lot
'It hurt me a lot here...'

D: sinexos?
continuously
'Continuously?'

P: enas sinexomenos ponos.
a continuous pain-NOM
'A continuous pain.'

D: exi eksarsis i etsi ine sinexja sinexja to iδio?
have-PRS:3SG peaks-ACC or like-this be-PRS:3SG continuously continuously the same-NOM
'Does it have peaks or is it the same all the time?'

P: tora exo ke tris meres pu me exi peθani ston pono. poli pono.
now have-PRS:1SG and three days-ACC that I-ACC have-PRS:3SG:IMPERS die-PFV in-the pain-ACC much pain-ACC
'I've been dying from pain for at least three days now. A lot of pain.'

D: toso poli.
so much
'So much.'

P: ine... kano kati enesis pu... prota.
be-PRS:3SG:IMPERS do-PRS:1SG some injections-ACC that before
'It is... I'm having some injections that... before.'

D: ne.
yes
'Yes.'

P: ...ke teliosane xθes to apoγevma.
and finish-PST:3PL yesterday the afternoon-ACC
'...and they finished yesterday afternoon.'

D: ne. kanate sinexja δilaδi kaθe teseris ores tis kanate?
yes do-IPFV:2PL continuously that-is every four hours-ACC they-ACC do-IPFV:2PL
'Yes. Were you having (them) continuously, that is, were you having one every four hours?'

P: tis kaname.
they-ACC do-IPFV:1PL
'We were.'

D: ipoδoria, pu tis kanate, eδo?
subcutaneously where they-ACC do-IPFV:2PL here
'Subcutaneously, where did you have them, here?'

P: eδo sto xeri.
here in-the arm-ACC
'Here, in the arm.'

D: to vlepo oti exi…
it-ACC see-PRS:1SG that have-PRS:3SG
'I can see that it has…'

P: sta xeria…
in-the arms-ACC
'In the arms…'

D: ne. sas epjanan kaθolu aftes?
yes you-ACC affect-IPFV:3PL at-all these-NOM
'Yes. Did they have any effect on you at all?'

P: me pjanane.
I-ACC affect-IPFV:3PL
'They had some effect on me.'

D: ja poso?
for how-long
'For how long?'

P: ja δio ores.
for two hours-ACC
'For two hours.'

D: ja ores e?
for hours-ACC eh
'For hours, eh?'

P: tris…
three-ACC
'Three…'

D: mmm... eee ston evangelizmo ipate isaste? sas evlepan eki sto iatrio ponu?
mmm eh at-the Evangelismos-ACC say-PST:2PL be-IPFV:2PL you-ACC see-IPFV:2PL there at-the clinic-ACC pain-GEN
'Mmm...eh did you say that you were at Evangelismos (Hospital)? Did you consult (them at) the pain management clinic, there?'

R: ixe pai.
have-PST:3SG go-PFV
'He had been (there).'

P: ixa pai mja fora.
have-PST:1SG go-PFV one time-ACC
'I had been (there) once.'

D: mono. ke tin aγoγi apo eki δilaδi sas tin kanonizan afti i o jatros...?
only and the treatment-ACC from there that-is you-GEN it-ACC regulate-IPFV:3PL they-NOM or the doctor-NOM
'That was all. So, was your treatment prescribed there (at the pain management clinic) by them or by the doctor...?'

P: o jatros.
the doctor-NOM
'(By) The doctor.'

D: ...o θerapon. ne.
the treating-NOM yes
'...the one who was responsible for my treatment. Yes.'

P: sto ongolojiko.
in-the oncological-ACC
'In the oncological clinic.'

D: ne. mmm. eee...
yes mmm eh
'Yes. Mmm. Eh...'

P: o x...
the man-NOM
'X...'

R: e, afu tora...
eh since now
'Eh, since now...'

D: na sas po… kala. ja na δume akrivos ti θa… kimaste to vraδi i sas ksipnai o ponos?
to-PARTCL you-GEN tell-PFV:NON-PST:1SG well just to-PARTCL see-PFV:NON-PST:1PL exactly what will sleep-PRS:2PL the night-ACC or you-ACC wake-up-PRS:3SG the pain-NOM
'Let me tell you… Well. Let's see exactly what we'll… Do you sleep at night or does the pain wake you up?'

P: δen kimame. δen exo kimiθi. δen exo kaθisi kaθolu… piso apo to… δilaδi δen boro na ksaploso etsi sto krevati δen boro na ksaploso sto spiti.
not sleep-PRS:1SG not have-PRS:1SG sleep-PFV not have-PRS:1SG sit-PFV at-all behind from the-ACC that-is not can-PRS:1SG to-PARTCL lie-down-PFV:NON-PST:1SG like-this on-the bed-ACC not can-PRS:1SG to-PARTCL lie-down-PFV:NON-PST:1SG in-the home-ACC
'I don't sleep. I haven't slept. I haven't sat at all… behind the… That is to say, I can't lie down on the bed like this, I can't lie down at home.'

D: mmm… perpatate?
mmm walk-PRS:2PL
'Mmm… Can you walk?'

P: na perpatiso, perpatao ala siγa, ponao.
to-PARTCL walk-PFV:NON-PST:1SG walk-PRS:1SG but slowly hurt-PRS:1SG
'To walk, I walk but slowly, I hurt.'

D: ponai?
hurt-PRS:3SG:IMPERS
'Does it hurt?'

R: i ke olo kaθistos etsi mazemenos jati ponai.
or and all seated-NOM like-this crouched-NOM because hurt-PRS:3SG
'Or even seated all the time, crouched like this, because he hurts.'

P: mazemenos…
crouched-NOM
'Crouched…'

D: trote kaθolu?
eat-PRS:2PL at-all
'Do you eat anything?'

P: zumera fajita.
juicy food-ACC
'Juicy food.'

D: otan fuskonete ke ponate…
when distend-PRS:2PL and hurt-PRS:2PL
'When you distend and hurt…'

P: ee, oxi. oxi eγo θelo na troo, meta apo to fajito ponao.
eh no no I-NOM want-PRS:1SG to-PARTCL eat-PRS:1SG after from the food-ACC hurt-PRS:1SG
'Eh, no. No, I do want to eat, it is after eating that I hurt.'

D: ne.
yes
'Yes.'

P: ponao poli.
hurt-PRS:1SG a-lot
'I hurt a lot.'

D: mmm… endaksi.
mmm all-right
'Mmm… All right.'

Name index

A
Aaron, David 180, 200
Aldrich, Sarah 4, 9, 134–136, 151, 156, 174, 197, 199
Antonopoulou, Eleni 153, 197, 202
Ashburn, Michael A. 9, 197
Athanasiadou, Angeliki 10, 197

B
Bacchini, Simone 14, 197
Badley, Elizabeth M. 9, 203
Bamberg, Michael 10, 197
Bastiaanse, Roelien 72, 200, 201
Baszanger, Isabelle 9, 197
Biber, Douglas 34, 197
Bloom, Lois 24, 197
Borsook, David 9, 115, 134, 175, 197
Brodwin, Paul E. 198, 200
Brugman, Claudia 143, 197

C
Cameron, Lynne 33, 137, 197, 198, 199, 200
Carlsson, Sven G. 18, 119, 134–135, 175, 200
Conrad, Susan 31, 197
Craig, Kenneth D. 18, 203
Crowdy, Steve 33, 197

D
Damasio, Antonio R. 10, 16–18, 197
Danielson, Ella 66, 134–135, 145, 203
Davidoff, Jules 72, 198
De Beaugrande, Robert 33, 198
De Bleser, Ria 72–73, 185, 198
Deignan, Alice 31, 33, 135, 137, 197, 198
Del Veccio Good, Mary-Jo 198, 200
DeSouza, Lorraine H. 113, 115, 117–118, 123, 136, 175, 198
Dirven, René 10, 197, 198, 200, 203
Drachman, Gaberell 80, 198

E
Eccleston, Chris 4, 9, 134–136, 151, 156, 174, 197
Edwards, Lindsey C. 9, 35, 198
Ekman, Paul 10, 198
Enfield, Nick J. 10–13, 19, 198
Engel, George 22, 198

F
Fabrega, Horatio Jr 9, 16, 18, 27, 119–120, 123–124, 133, 136, 153, 198
Fernandez, Ephrem 118–119, 123, 134–135, 198
Foolen, Ad 18, 26, 59–61, 101, 139, 179, 194, 198
Foucault, Michel 9, 66, 199
Frank, Andrew O. 113, 115, 117–118, 123, 136, 175, 198
Freud, Sigmund 17–18, 199
Fries, Peter. H. 80, 199, 200

G
Gaston-Johansson, Fannie 9, 199, 203
Gavriilidou, Zoe 117, 203
Georgoudis, George 9, 114–115, 199
Gergen, Kenneth J. 66, 199
Ghadessy, Mohsen 80, 198, 199, 202
Gibbon, Daffyd 34–35, 199
Gibbs, Raymond W. 133–134, 199
Goldstein, Irwin 19–20, 22, 199
Good, Byron J. 9, 35, 49, 198, 200
Greenberg, Joseph H. 80, 199
Gustafson, Donald F. 2–3, 18, 25, 28, 45, 199
Gwyn, Richard 135–156, 200

H
Haiman, John 141, 200
Hallberg, Lillemor R.-M. 18, 119, 134–135, 175, 200
Halliday, Michael Alexander Kirkwood 1–2, 3–6, 8, 14, 27–29, 31, 34, 37–39, 44–45, 48, 61, 73, 75, 77–78, 80–81, 85, 91–92, 95–97, 99, 101, 103–106, 108, 110–111, 114, 123–124, 126–127, 129–132, 134, 144–145, 151, 184, 186–187, 189–190, 200
Harre, Rom 66, 200
Hasan, Ruqaiya 80, 199, 200
Hatzidaki, Ourania 3, 14, 25, 27, 34, 46, 60, 72, 184, 188, 200, 202
Heywood, John 135, 153, 204
Holmes, Janet 34, 200
Holton, David 117, 200
Horrocks, Geoffrey 80, 200

I
Inchaurralde, Carlos 47, 200
Izard, Carroll E. 10, 200

J
Jackendoff, Ray 180, 200
Jackson, Jean 9, 19, 200
Janal, Malvin N. 9, 200
Johnson, Mark 1, 4, 7, 13, 133, 201
Jones, Roger B. 23, 200
Jonkers, Roel 72, 200, 201

K
Kauschke, Christina 72–73, 185, 198

Kenny, Anthony John Patrick 3, 25, 201
Kern, Steven E. 136, 201
Kidron, Yael 173, 201
Kim, Mikyong 73, 201
Kleinman, Arthur 9, 198, 200, 201
Kövecses, Zoltán 1, 4, 7, 10–11, 13, 104, 131, 133–134, 137–138, 144, 147–148, 150–151, 156–160, 165, 173, 178–179, 191, 193, 201
Kripke, Saul A. 3, 22, 24, 187, 201
Kugelmann, Robert 4, 9, 19, 134–136, 145, 167, 201
Kuzar, Ron 173, 201

L
Lakoff, George 1, 4, 7, 13, 66, 131, 133, 144, 200, 201
Langacker, Ronald 38, 142–43, 201
Lange, K. L. 73, 204
Lascaratou, Chryssoula 2–4, 14, 25–27, 46, 60, 72, 80, 82, 103, 136, 138, 141, 145, 150–151, 155–156, 161, 169, 178, 180, 184, 188, 191–192, 195, 197, 201, 202, 204
LeBel, Alyssa A. 9, 115, 134, 175, 197
Leder, Drew 145, 202
LeDoux, Joseph 10, 18, 202
Levin, Beth 97, 202
Levinas, Emmanuel 9, 202

M
Mackridge, Peter 117, 200
Marmaridou, Sophia 2–4, 14, 26, 60, 103, 136, 138, 141–142, 145, 150–151, 155–156, 161, 169, 178, 180, 191–192, 195, 202
Masterson, Jackie 72, 198
Matthiessen, Christian 61, 80, 187, 202
McBurney, Donald H. 35, 202
McCaffery, Margo 16, 202
McPeek, Bucknam 9, 115, 134, 175, 197
Melzack, Ronald 9, 15, 66, 113–114, 118, 134, 202, 203, 205
Merskey, Harold 15, 20, 23, 203
Moore, Roger 34–35, 199
Morris, David B. 9, 203
Moser, Amalia 51, 143, 203

N
Nakas, Thanassis 117, 203
Niemeier, Susanne 10, 13, 197, 198, 200, 203
Nikiforidou, Kiki 51, 143, 202, 203, 204, 205
Nissenbaum, Helen Fay 10, 203
Norberg, Astrid 4, 9, 119–120, 134–136, 153, 172, 175, 204
Norvell, Kristine Turner 9, 203

O
Oldham, Jacqueline A. 9, 114, 199
Omondi, Lucia N. 10, 203

P
Papageorgiou, Ann C. 9, 203
Paulson, Margareta 66, 134–135, 145, 203
Pavlenko, Aneta 10–11, 76, 203
Pearce, Shirley A. 9, 35, 198, 203
Perrott, Alisa 9, 203
Peters, Hans 150, 155, 203
Philippaki-Warburton, Irene 80, 200, 203
Pincus, Tamar 9, 203
Poole, Garry D. 18, 203

R
Rappaport Hovav, Malka 97, 202
Reppen, Randi 31, 197
Rey, Roselyn 9, 203
Rice, Linda J. 9, 197
Rosaldo, Michelle Z. 11, 204

S
Scarry, Elaine 9, 19, 161, 195–196, 204
Schneider, Sandra L. 73, 204
Schweizer, Harold 9, 195, 204
Semino, Elena 135, 153, 204
Shapiro, Lewis P. 73, 204
Short, Mick 34, 114–115, 135, 153, 190, 199, 204
Sinclair, John McHardy 31, 34, 204
Smith, M. C. 135, 203, 204
Söderberg, Siv 4, 9, 66, 119–120, 134–136, 153, 172, 175, 203, 204
Solomon, Robert C. 10, 204
Sontag, Susan 135, 153, 156, 204

T
Tabakowska, Elzbieta 10, 197
Talmy, Len 1, 4, 7, 13, 104, 138, 156–158, 169, 178, 192, 204
Theodoropoulou, Maria 11, 204
Theophanopoulou-Kontou, Dimitra 51, 143, 204
Thomas, Jenny 32, 204
Thompson, Cynthia K. 73, 201, 204
Toombs, Kay S. 9, 204
Torgerson, Warren S. 9, 15, 113, 118–119, 134, 202
Towery, Stuart 118–119, 123, 134–135, 198
Tsimpli, Ianthi-Maria 80, 204
Tyma, Stephen 9, 16, 18, 27, 119–120, 123–124, 133, 136, 153, 198
Tzartzanos, Achileas 80, 204
Tzavaras, Thanasis 175, 205

V
Veloudis, Ioannis 51, 143, 205

W
Waddie, Nicola A. 9, 20, 205
Wall, Patrick D. 9, 203, 205
Walters, A. 15, 205
Watson, Jean 135, 205
Watson, Paul J. 9, 114, 199
Wierzbicka, Anna 5, 10–13, 19, 39, 47–48, 57, 76–77, 184–185, 198, 205
Wilson, Andrew 32, 204
Winski, Richard 34–35, 199
Wittgenstein, Ludwig 2–3, 5, 9, 19–25, 28–29, 65, 101, 186, 188, 195, 200, 201, 205

Z
Zimmerman, Lani 9, 203

Subject index

A
acute pain 66–68
affective pain descriptors 115–116, 120, 122–123
agency 42–43, 78, 89, 97, 161
agentivity 155–156, 192
Agonist 156–158, 160–161, 167, 169, 171–174, 193
animacy 155–156, 192
Antagonist 156–158, 160–161, 163, 167, 169, 171–174, 193
assessment of pain 114–115, 118, 123, 166, 189–190
authentic communicative situation 34
  see also authentic dialogues
authentic dialogues 3, 5, 122, 190
  see also naturally occurring language data
automatic pain reactions 6, 26, 60–61, 73, 78, 101, 139, 183

B
body 1, 6–7, 13, 15–16, 18, 20, 66, 85, 88, 100–101, 104, 110–111, 113, 120, 124, 136, 138, 145–146, 149–155, 165, 174, 178–180, 184, 186, 188–189, 192–194
  part 4, 6, 48, 50, 52, 55, 62–66, 70–71, 74, 80, 88–91, 95–97, 111, 187–189
bottom-up approach 32, 138

C
cancer 32, 153, 156
causal chain 159–160, 163, 166–167, 171, 178
causes of pain 7, 15, 31, 64–65, 92, 119, 131, 148, 156–161, 163, 165–167, 170–171, 178, 180, 184, 187, 190, 192–194
chronic pain 66–68, 108, 113, 123, 167, 175, 187, 189
cognitive semantics 1–2, 4, 7, 11–13, 19, 66, 103, 126, 131, 178, 183, 191
continuum 6, 8, 25–26, 60, 78, 90, 101, 124, 139, 184, 194–195
  see also spectrum
  expressive-descriptive axis of
    see expressive-descriptive axis of continuum
control 76, 139, 143, 147, 155, 158, 160, 169–173, 179, 192, 194
corpus 1, 3, 5, 14, 31–34, 46, 48, 50, 55–56, 61, 136–137, 140, 156, 179, 183–184, 188, 191, 193
  see also subcorpus
  linguistics 31, 136–137
  of Greek Texts (CGT) 105, 116
cry / cries 6, 19, 21, 24–26, 48, 59–61, 65, 78, 101, 188, 194
  see also primitive cry
  of complaint 24, 65, 85, 186, 195

D
definition of pain 4, 13, 15–16, 59
doctor-patient discourse 5, 7, 45, 180, 193
  see also medical discourse
  interaction 139–140, 145, 151, 155, 159, 178–179, 193

E
effects of pain 7, 104, 148–149, 160–161, 163, 165–167, 169, 179, 184, 193
  confining effect 167
    see also meta-effect
  meta-effect 159, 167, 170
  paralysing effect 169
    see also meta-effect
embodiment 7, 104, 138, 165, 179, 193
emotion and metaphor 13, 104, 126, 131, 133–135, 137–138, 144, 147–148, 150, 152, 156–160, 165, 168–169, 171, 173, 178, 193
emotional aspect of pain 4, 13, 15–16, 18, 35, 59, 144, 150, 159–160, 169, 172
evaluative word 114
exclamations of pain 21, 23, 52–53, 57, 78, 85, 101, 186, 194
  see also interjections of pain
expressive-descriptive axis of continuum 6, 78, 101, 184, 194
external manifestations of pain 18, 23, 159–160
  responses of pain 157, 166–167, 170–171

F
force dynamic (image) schema 4, 7, 104, 138, 149, 156–158, 161, 169–170, 172, 178, 184, 192
function of pain language
  descriptive function 6, 8, 26, 59, 101, 139, 195
    see also description
  dual function 24–25, 184, 195
  expressive function 6, 24–26, 59, 61, 65, 85, 101, 186, 194–195
    see also expression
    gradience of, *see* gradience of expressive function
Functional Grammar 1, 5, 27, 29, 37

G
gradience of expressive function 6, 101, 194

Greek Short Form of McGill Pain Questionnaire (GR-SFMPQ), *see* McGill Pain Questionnaire (MPQ)
groans 6, 19, 26, 48, 60–61, 78, 101, 194

H
holistic
configuration 6, 88, 100, 179, 187–188
construal 80–81, 188
experience 26, 90, 140, 145
expression 78, 92, 99, 179
thematic perspective 6, 82, 186

I
illness 20, 66, 135, 145–146, 156,
image-schema 13, 149
container image-schema 150–152
force image-schema, *see* force dynamic (image) schema
source – path – goal image-schema 152
image schematic (conceptual) structure 155, 178, 183
impersonal constructions 6, 27, 42, 57, 61, 63, 65, 70–73, 84–85, 99–101, 130, 185–188, 194
intensity of pain 6, 113–118, 122–124, 129, 147–149, 161, 165–166, 180, 186, 189–190, 192
interjections of pain 6, 48, 57, 61, 65, 78, 101, 186, 194
International Association for the Study of Pain (IASP) 4, 13, 15, 31, 59
involvement of the sufferer's self 1, 5, 46–48, 141, 176, 183–184, 187–188

L
language of emotions 4, 5, 10–13, 19, 26, 47–48, 57, 59–60, 75–77, 139, 179, 184–185, 194
languages
English 1, 3, 5, 10, 12, 14, 27, 29, 37–38, 40, 42, 47–48, 61–62, 72–73, 75–77, 80, 83, 92, 94–97, 99, 104, 108, 110–111, 118–120, 122–125, 127, 130–133, 144, 150, 155, 166, 184, 186–187, 190
German 72
Greek 1–8, 26, 28–29, 34, 37, 40, 42, 44–48, 50, 55, 57, 59, 61–62, 67, 71–77, 80, 82–83, 91–92, 94–97, 99–101, 103–105, 110–111, 113–116, 118, 120, 122–125, 127, 129–132, 134–136, 138–140, 142, 147, 153, 155–156, 158, 160–161, 165–167, 169, 178, 183–191, 193–195
Russian 47–48, 76–77, 184–185
Swedish 120, 136
location of pain 55–57, 64, 83–84, 88, 96, 100, 104, 111, 124, 150–151, 153, 179, 187, 189
locus of pain, *see* location of pain

M
McGill Pain Questionnaire (MPQ) 113–115, 123, 166, 190
Greek Short Form of McGill Pain Questionnaire (GR-SFMPQ) 114–116, 118, 122–123, 190
measurement of pain 6, 115, 189–190
medical discourse 32–33
metaphor
event structure metaphor 144, 147, 152–153, 157, 173
general metaphor 7, 104, 131, 138, 144, 157, 168, 171, 173, 178, 193
generic-level metaphor 157, 184
generic-level master metaphor 104, 178, 193
master metaphor 4, 157
ontological metaphor 140, 145, 150–151, 153, 155–156, 173, 192
specific-level metaphors 7, 104, 138, 157–158, 164, 173, 178, 184, 193
metonymy 7, 13, 119, 165, 179, 193
metonymic basis 119, 165
metonymic process 164, 166
metonymic relationship 119, 165, 190
metonymic vehicle 165
metonymically applied source domains 148, 166
metonymically conceptualised aspects of pain 161, 163, 166
metonymically derived metaphors 113, 119, 165–166, 180, 190, 194

N
Natural Semantic Metalanguage (NSM) 12–13
see also universal semantic primitives
naturally occurring language data 5, 31–32, 137, 183, 189
neuroscience 5, 10, 16–18

O
objectification of pain 26, 60, 107, 129–130, 139–143, 145, 147, 151, 155, 178–180, 192, 195

P
pain
assessment of, *see* assessment of pain
causes of, *see* causes of pain
definition of, *see* definition of pain
effects of, *see* effects of pain
emotional aspect of, *see* emotional aspect of pain
exclamations of, *see* exclamations of pain
external manifestations of, *see* external manifestations of pain
external responses of, *see* external responses of pain
intensity of, *see* intensity of pain
interjections of, *see* interjections of pain
location of, *see* location of pain
locus of, *see* locus of pain
measurement of, *see* measurement of pain
objectification of, *see* objectification of pain
personification of, *see* personification of pain
qualities of, *see* qualities of pain

sensory aspect of, *see* sensory aspect of pain
sensory effects of, *see* sensory effects of pain
(un)boundedness of, *see* (un) boundedness of pain
pain as
circumstance 29, 38, 46, 96, 111, 131, 166, 170–172, 178, 184, 192
force 4, 7, 104, 116, 138, 140, 148–150, 152–153, 155–161, 163, 165, 167, 169–173, 178, 180, 184, 192–194
possession 6, 51, 55, 105–107, 124–126, 136, 142–146, 189, 191–192
see also pain as relational: attributive: possessive process
process
behavioural process 78, 83
existential process 83, 85, 90, 100, 130
material process 55, 78, 82, 85, 89, 91–93, 95–96, 98–99, 127, 132, 141, 155, 166, 172, 188
mental process 55, 91, 95–96, 99–100, 128, 141, 185
meteorological process 42, 85, 186–187
relational: attributive process 55, 74–75, 77, 88, 97, 128, 132, 141, 144
relational: attributive: possessive process 55, 125–127, 142–145
verbal process 131–132
pain behaviour 9, 18–19, 24, 59, 61, 194
pain descriptors 113–114, 118–123, 166, 189–190
see also affective pain descriptors, sensory pain descriptors, evaluative word
participants in pain constructions
Actor / Agent 166, 170, 172
Actor 78, 89–90, 93, 95, 98, 127, 132, 147, 153, 155, 192
Agent 78, 89, 91–93, 95, 97, 98, 100, 127, 132, 155, 169, 188
Attribute 74–76, 88, 97, 125, 128, 132, 141, 147, 191
Behaver 78, 83, 188
Beneficiary 127
Carrier 43, 74–75, 88, 125, 128–129, 132, 188, 191
Existent 83, 130, 191
Goal 93, 95, 98, 127, 132, 155, 172, 188, 190
Identified 129, 191
Identifier 129, 191
Location 131
Medium 42, 83, 85, 90
Phenomenon 91–92, 95–96, 99–100, 128, 141, 191
Sayer 131–132
Senser 75, 91, 95–96, 99–100, 128, 141, 188
Setting 83, 88, 90, 100, 188
Token 129, 191
Value 129
personal constructions 4, 6, 26, 62–65, 70–72, 185–186
personification of pain 111, 136, 141, 153, 155–156, 161, 173, 178–180, 189, 192–193
primitive cry 26, 65, 139, 186
primitive reactions 19, 25, 60

Q
qualities of pain 6, 15, 108, 113–115, 118–120, 122–124, 129, 161, 165–166, 180, 189–190, 192, 194

R
reflexive patterns 76, 95–96
repression 17

S
screams 6, 26, 48, 60–61, 78, 101, 194
sensory aspect of pain 15, 59, 113–114, 118–119, 148, 165, 175, 190
see also sensory effects of pain
sensory effects of pain 7, 104, 148, 165–166, 179, 184, 193
sensory pain descriptors 115, 119–120, 123, 190
separatist view 10
skeletal scenario
see skeletal structure
skeletal structure 158–160, 171
source domains of pain metaphors 117, 119, 126, 131, 135, 144, 147–150, 152–153, 158, 164–165, 190
spectrum 26, 60
subcorpus 3, 46, 53, 56, 136

T
tissue damage 7, 15–16, 31, 104, 119, 138, 148, 163–166, 179, 184, 193
top-down approach 138
transitivity 37–39, 41–43, 61, 78
intransitive constructions 4, 6–7, 26–27, 39–40, 42–43, 61–65, 69–73, 75–78, 82, 89, 101, 132, 140, 147, 154, 178–179, 183, 185–188, 192, 194
transitive constructions 7, 39–40, 42–44, 62–63, 65, 70–73, 82, 92–93, 128, 132, 140, 147, 155, 172, 178, 183, 185, 192

U
(un)boundedness of pain 104–106, 124, 128, 131, 145, 147, 168, 189, 192
universal aspects of human physiology of pain 13, 104, 119, 138, 148, 165–166, 179–180, 184, 193–194
universal semantic primitives 11
see also Natural Semantic Metalanguage (NSM)
universalist approach 10

In the series *Converging Evidence in Language and Communication Research* the following titles have been published thus far or are scheduled for publication:

10 **STEEN, Gerard J.:** Finding Metaphor in Grammar and Usage. A methodological analysis of theory and research. xiv, 425 pp. + index. *Expected November 2007*

9 **LASCARATOU, Chryssoula:** The Language of Pain. Expression or description. 2007. xii, 237 pp.

8 **PLÜMACHER, Martina and Peter HOLZ (eds.):** Speaking of Colors and Odors. 2007. vi, 244 pp.

7 **SHARIFIAN, Farzad and Gary B. PALMER (eds.):** Applied Cultural Linguistics. Implications for second language learning and intercultural communication. 2007. xiv, 170 pp.

6 **DEIGNAN, Alice:** Metaphor and Corpus Linguistics. 2005. x, 236 pp.

5 **JOHANSSON, Sverker:** Origins of Language. Constraints on hypotheses. 2005. xii, 346 pp.

4 **KERTÉSZ, András:** Cognitive Semantics and Scientific Knowledge. Case studies in the cognitive science of science. 2004. viii, 261 pp.

3 **LOUWERSE, Max and Willie van PEER (eds.):** Thematics. Interdisciplinary Studies. 2002. x, 448 pp.

2 **ALBERTAZZI, Liliana (ed.):** Meaning and Cognition. A multidisciplinary approach. 2000. vi, 270 pp.

1 **HORIE, Kaoru (ed.):** Complementation. Cognitive and functional perspectives. 2000. vi, 242 pp.